I0824157

Praise for *One Scan Saved My Life*

"Shira's story is one of courage, awareness, and the power of acting before it's too late."

—**Tony Robbins**, #1 *New York Times* bestselling author and the world's #1 life and business strategist

"Shira's experience is one that too many people have gone through. She is brave for being so open about her lung cancer experience, because this is how you bring awareness and help to change policy in our country."

—**Andy Slavitt**, USofCare Co-Founder and President Obama's Head of Medicare and Medicaid

"Even as a trained lung surgeon, I find cases like young Shira Boehler's shocking. Her riveting story should be grasped by all."

—**Dr. Mehmet Oz**, nationally recognized thoracic surgeon and President Trump's Head of Medicare and Medicaid

"As a physician and chief medical officer, nothing makes me happier than helping our patients. Shira is so amazing and I feel lucky to have been a small part of her journey. Her experience will change things for so many."

—**Ben Kornitzer**, CMO of Aetna

"Shira's story is the perfect example of why we created Function and Ezra. We are excited to amplify her story and work together to save more lives."

—**Jonathan Swerdlin**, Co-Founder and CEO of Function Health

"With the rise of early onset cancers, there needs to be a reconsideration of conventional screening guidelines and an expansion of the definition of 'high risk.' 'Early detection saves lives' is a mantra we live by in medicine; it is incumbent on the medical community as well as policy makers to ensure that we are capturing as many survivable cancers as possible."

—**Dr. Natalie Azar**, medical contributor for NBC News and assistant clinical professor of medicine and rheumatology at NYU Langone

"In this deeply personal and moving memoir, Shira Boehler shares her journey through a shocking, unexpected diagnosis of lung cancer, shattering the myth that this disease affects only smokers, men, and older people. This invaluable book, animated by her powerful advocacy, provides a critical call to action for more widely available early detection methods, the urgent need to focus on understudied sex differences in the disease, and increased public awareness. Her message: Scientific research, cutting-edge technology, and expanded screening will save lives."

— **Rear Admiral Susan Blumenthal, MD**, (ret.) First Deputy Assistant Secretary for Women's Health and former US Assistant Surgeon General

One Scan Saved My Life

How One Woman's Story Will Change the Way We Detect Lung Cancer

Shira Kupperman Boehler

Foreword by Anne Wojcicki & Janet M. Wojcicki

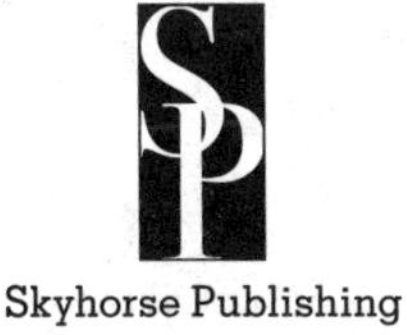

Skyhorse Publishing

Skyhorse Publishing books may be purchased in bulk at special discounts for sales promotion, corporate gifts, fund-raising, or educational purposes. Special editions can also be created to specifications. For details, contact the Special Sales Department, Skyhorse Publishing, 307 Fifth Avenue, 4th Floor, New York, NY 10016 or info@skyhorsepublishing.com.

Visit our website at www.skyhorsepublishing.com and the author's website at www.cancerdoesntcare.com

Please follow our publisher Tony Lyons on Instagram @tonylyonsisuncertain and author Shira Boehler on Instagram @shiraboehler.

10 9 8 7 6 5 4 3 2

Library of Congress Cataloging-in-Publication Data is available on file.

Cover design by David Ter-Avanesyan
Cover image credit courtesy of the author

Print ISBN: 978-1-5107-8802-2
Ebook ISBN: 978-1-5107-8803-9

Printed in the United States of America

Contents

This book is dedicated to my husband, who insisted I get the scan that saved my life; to my children, who helped me find laughter in the hardest moments; to my parents, to Kim, and to all of my doctors who have devoted their lives to fighting this disease; and to those who lost their lives to lung cancer, as well as those we will find early enough to survive, as I have.

If this book inspires you to share your story, I invite you to post it on my website by scanning the QR code below or visiting www.cancerdoesntcare.com.

Foreword

When Shira called us and told us she had been diagnosed with lung cancer we were shocked—but unfortunately not as shocked as we should have been, since our sister Susan had just recently passed away from lung cancer at the age of 54.

I (Anne) have known Shira since my early 20s and our lives have woven in and out of each other's spheres. We all reconnected during the pandemic, when we had the good fortune of living near each other. Shira was a bright spot in a world that had gone dark. She was enthusiastic, always happy to tell a joke, and loved seeing her kids run around and enjoy their freedom. Shira is energy.

When Shira told us she had lung cancer, we knew there were one of two paths in her future: Lung cancer that is contained, is resectable, and has high survival rates. Or lung cancer that has spread, has a poor prognosis. When our sister was diagnosed with lung cancer, it had already spread to her hip and bones. We prayed during her bone biopsy that the cancer was a treatable lymphoma, but it was not. We remember the shock of this diagnosis and cried uncontrollably after her biopsy. We felt compeltely powerless. The future was defined.

Susan was diagnosed with stage 4 non-small cell lung cancer at age 54—as a person with no tobacco use history. We realized that there was no clear way the United States health system, Susan's doctors, or our family could have done much to prevent this terminal diagnosis. This was particularly devastating, as my sister Janet and I have dedicated our professional lives to health prevention and promotion. Janet is a Professor of Pediatrics and Epidemiology at the University of California San Francisco, and I am the founder and CEO of 23andMe Research Institute. For us, prevention of disease is a mantra that we live and breathe.

Why hadn't Susan been screened for lung cancer? It is the most common cause of cancer death among women in the United States (accounting for 21 percent of all female cancer deaths in the United States), and yet she had never been approached for a lung cancer screening. Susan had been meticulous in her regular screening mammographies for breast cancer and colonoscopies and fecal immunochemical tests (FIT) for colorectal cancer, and yet cancer deaths from these other types of cancer represent only a fraction of those deaths from lung cancer. If she had known about the high mortality rate from lung cancer or had been offered any screening, she surely would have agreed.

Sadly, we are not alone in this unfortunate path and outcome that we traveled as a family. We have no universal screenings for Americans for lung cancer. As such, lung cancer is often diagnosed very late, at stage 4, when it has already spread (in 30 to 40 percent of new cases). When lung cancer is diagnosed so late, the prognosis is dismal and the health system is only doing catch-up on these patients, just like it was on our sister Susan.

But the story could have been vastly different if Susan's lung cancer was caught at stage 1, before metastasis. Susan's story could have been Shira's story if her cancer had been detected earlier.

Shira's story is scary, but it's a story of success. Shira's cancer was caught early, at stage 1, because she had access to lung cancer screening that saved her life, and her chance for long term survival is very high.

Shira's cancer was luckily caught early because she had access to MRI and low-dose CT imaging modalities. However, in the United States, we do not have a *universal lung cancer screening program* for the general population, or even a targeted screening program for those who have a family history of lung cancer or other risk factors, including exposure to radon or a moderate history of tobacco use. Medicare and private insurance companies will only reimburse for lung cancer screening (recommended to be a low-dose CT) for those 50 to 77 years if you have a 20+ pack year history (1 pack a day for 20 years or more) and are a current smoker or quit within the last 15 years. Even in this *extremely* high risk population, a shockingly low 2 to 6 percent of those who are eligible actually get the screening, in part due to low levels of awareness of screening guidelines, reimbursements and benefits among both patients and providers.

We can do better. We need to demand action by our government and policymakers to invest in lung cancer detection and make lung cancer a treatable disease for everyone. Our research and innovation capabilities as Americans are second to none, and we can turn the tide on lung cancer deaths by designing ways to make sure that there are universal lung cancer screening modalities, just as there are for breast and colorectal cancers. Shira, fortunately, had access to imaging that saved her life; but access to these lifesaving screening should not be limited to those with financial resources or awareness and knowledge.

Other countries are showing the United States how these low-dose CT programs can be implemented to save lives. Taiwan, for example, provides access to low-dose CT for all individuals with a first degree relative with a lung cancer diagnosis. Additionally, Taiwan lowered the age of eligibility for women to 45 years, given the increasing rate of lung cancer diagnosis among younger women. Poland, in Eastern Europe, was able to substantially increase uptake among those eligible in rural areas through the use of mobile CT units.

Americans have a history of scientific innovation and creativity. Our government and public health system have not (yet) focused these energies on preventing deaths from lung cancer. We are hopeful that Shira's courageous story and experience, told here with Susan's (and many others like her) in the background, will be a call to action to get our gears in motion and push for prevention and reform to save many lives. We believe that we have the technology and know-how right now and right here to change the trajectory of lung cancer mortality.

—Anne Wojcicki, Co-Founder and CEO of 23andMe, and Janet M. Wojcicki, PhD MPH MAS, Department of Pediatrics at the University of California, San Francisco

Introduction

On Monday, September 29, 2025, I received the most terrifying and unexpected news of my life: I had LUNG CANCER. I was only forty-three years old and had never smoked a single puff of a cigarette. I also exercised a few times a week, did my best to eat a balanced diet, and saw my doctors regularly. Yet, I still found myself sitting across from my doctor in the exam room being told that a scan showed a fast-growing, highly invasive tumor in my right lung. "What? No way!" I kept telling my doctor. "No way! Wrong person, wrong scan!"

Lung cancer should have killed me, but thanks to an early preventive scan, I am alive and well. The story of learning I had lung cancer and then beating it has taught me more than I ever thought I'd know about this deadly disease—and how science, technology, government, and most important, people like you and me hold the key to stopping it. Lung cancer is a misunderstood, over-stigmatized, underfunded, and under-researched disease that has grown into an urgent health crisis—especially for women—and there is no doubt in my mind that we can change that.

One scan saved my life, and I want that to be true for more people.

My world changed on a Monday morning that started just like any other. I woke up my four kids and got them dressed, downstairs, fed, and out the door. I loaded them up in the minivan, dropped them at school, and raced to the park to do my six-mile run before my doctor's appointment. I was living in Nashville, Tennessee, thinking I was a model of health, yet all that was about to change with my diagnosis.

Let's back up a second. This journey *actually* began on a work trip to New York a few months prior, when my husband, Adam, suggested I get a full-body preventive MRI for a baseline look at my general health. I gave him some major pushback. I am extremely claustrophobic and my annual breast MRI and mammogram are all that I can handle. I freak out in those machines, and I mean totally panic and freak out. My mother had breast cancer while I was in college and I am religious about getting scans . . . but I do them because I have to, not because I want to.

Adam and I battled for a bit, but he won, and I made an appointment for a full-body MRI on our trip. I squeezed my eyes shut, sang *The Little Mermaid* soundtrack on repeat in my head, and counted the minutes till I got out of that machine while my heart raced. In the end, it detected a "non-urgent, typically harmless" spot on the middle lobe of my right lung. My report recommended I follow up with my doctor if I developed any symptoms. *Fine, Adam,* I thought. *I did it, and I hope you are happy, because the MRI found nothing!*

When I got back to Nashville, I shared my MRI pictures with my radiologist friend Kim over a sushi lunch. She rolled her eyes, said MRIs were not the right way to look at lungs, and told me I could follow up with a CT scan for less than a thousand dollars out of pocket. She was not worried in the slightest, but—except for the fact I'd have to get into yet another machine—I didn't think there was much harm in investigating more. I had options.

It was the best decision of my life. My low-dose CT scan revealed a stage I lung adenocarcinoma that was growing so fast I needed surgery as soon as possible. I had no history, no symptoms, and met no risk factors, but was facing an aggressive lung cancer.

How did this happen?

I wish my story was unique, but it is not. In the United States today, lung cancer kills almost 125,000 people a year, and it is the leading killer among all types of cancer. In fact, lung cancer causes more deaths each year than breast cancer, pancreatic cancer, and ovarian cancer

COMBINED.[1] Like me, 25 percent of those diagnosed with lung cancer have never smoked a cigarette,[2] and this, among other factors, makes them ineligible for insurance coverage of early screening. By the time people like me develop symptoms, their cancer cells have likely spread to other organs, making it too late for a cure. While surgery, chemotherapy, radiation or other treatments can extend their life past a few months, it unfortunately can't save them. The fact remains that because lung cancer is typically caught in later, metastasized stages, it's a death sentence for almost everyone.

My dad is a lung doctor (crazy, right?), and he raised my brothers and me to fear cigarettes. "No smoking allowed. Smoking causes lung cancer and other bad diseases." As a pulmonologist, he ingrained this into us, so when I found out about my cancer, I was in even more shock. And as I shared my news, I learned that almost everyone I know assumes the same thing. My closest friends and colleagues—people I see daily—asked me if I smoked, when I quit, or how I hid my smoking addiction. What? I can't even tell you how many people assumed I was a smoker. The reality is that society thinks of lung cancer as a "deserved" disease. If you get it, you obviously brought it on yourself by smoking.

This is far from true. According to the American Lung Association, smoking rates have fallen by 73 percent among adults since 1965, but lung cancer rates have not, especially among women under fifty. Many doctors and scientists studying this disease believe that we are in the middle of a women's health crisis, but no one has taken ownership of lung cancer the way that they've tackled other "women's diseases" like breast, cervical, and ovarian cancers. Before my diagnosis, I'd never heard of a lung cancer march, fundraising campaign, or month dedicated to awareness (it's November, by the way). I wasn't sure who lung cancer affected, how it was treated, or where research into it stands. And I didn't know about lung cancer screenings and why insurance pays for some people to get them but doesn't cover most.

Now I do, and it's what I want to share with you.

Only in the last twenty years have federal guidelines recommended lung cancer screenings with a low-dose CT (LDCT) scan for high-risk patients, meaning Americans fifty to eighty years of age who smoke or—in the past fifteen years—have smoked the equivalent of a pack a day for twenty years. Hmmm . . . remember when I said a quarter of those who die from lung cancer are never-smokers? These guidelines are clearly inadequate. Early screening is not perfect, but the data is clear: LDCTs reduce lung cancer mortality rates by 20 percent.[3] Why are we not screening more? We are pushed to get mammograms at forty, colonoscopies at forty-five, and Pap smears starting in our twenties. So why not a lung scan, too?

In the short time since my life was saved by a lung scan, I've jumped headfirst into answering this urgent question. I've dug into the research, science, and guidelines, learning all the reasons why I and others have gotten lung cancer. I have spoken with dozens of doctors and experts about the anatomy of the disease, the risk factors for it, the innovations shaping its future, and the treatments that can cure it, and I've met with countless advocates about the critical need for early detection. I've become friends with surgeons, scientists, and patients like me, and—happily—I have even met a few other lung cancer survivors. (Before I had cancer, I didn't even think about whether there *were* lung cancer survivors.) All these stories, findings, science, and recommendations are here on these pages, told through the lens of my unexpected journey. This book is my effort to raise awareness, educate, and give others hope in the fight against lung cancer. Because there *is* hope.

I want to acknowledge again how lucky I am. I was screened, caught the disease early, and had successful surgery right away. My lymph nodes were clear, meaning the cancer hadn't spread, and I went home to my husband and kids with only a cough, a few scars, and stories I'll tell for the rest of my life. Others have not been so fortunate. Thanks to science, surgery, and early detection, lung cancer did not kill me, but it has changed my life. I wish the same was true for every other lung cancer patient.

Lung cancer is all too often treated as a problem that can't or won't ever be solved. I'm determined to change that. In the past fifty years, we've successfully brought lung cancer diagnosis and mortality rates down by a huge margin, but there is so much more work to do. I wasn't a statistic, and you and your loved ones should not be either.

We need scans and other cancer screening tests to be recommended and covered. We need to change the narrative around lung cancer. We need to recognize that it is not just a smoker's disease. We need to see this as a female health crisis, a young person's health crisis. We're all in this fight together. I hope you will join me.

Chapter One
The Spot

Summer 2025

Adam and I were in New York City for work. We had back-to-back meetings over a quick thirty-six-hour period, and I wanted to find time to see a few friends, too.

"Shira, why don't you get a whole-body MRI scan while we're here? I did one last year. Let's do it together this year."

Adam's heart was in the right place, but there was no way I was saying yes. Fine, I understood that a whole-body MRI might find potential problems like cancer, aneurysms, fatty liver, and gallstones, but I also knew it meant being trapped on my back in a small, dark tube for an hour. My claustrophobia made me put my guard up. Hard pass!

"Nope, sorry," I said to Adam. "I know you did it, but I cannot put myself through that torture, nor will I."

About seven months earlier, Adam had paid out-of-pocket for an advanced, full-body MRI. MRI stands for Magnetic Resonance Imaging, and it's a scan that uses magnet radio waves and a computer to create detailed images of your internal organs. MRIs do not use radiation, and testing involves lying on your back inside a closed structure while the machine's magnetic field works with computer-generated radio waves to scan throughout your body. Adam's MRI revealed he had an asymptomatic sinus blockage (silent sinusitis syndrome) that could, in time, cause the bones in his cheeks and eye orbit to erode, so he decided to have surgery to correct it. Now it was summer, the problem was in the past, and Adam was breathing free and easy. An MRI had helped him dodge a bullet, and it made total sense that he would want the same for me.

"Shira," Adam pressed, "look what it found for me. I know you are healthy, but don't you think establishing a baseline in our forties is a good idea?"

I knew he was right, but I just couldn't do it. "The idea of being in that tube terrifies me," I said. "I'd do it if there was a problem, but there's *no* problem."

"I'm sure there's not," he continued, "but an MRI discovered this little, weird thing in my sinuses that I wouldn't have found until it became an issue. I dealt with it early, before it got worse, and I'm glad I did. I promise the MRI isn't bad. You can watch a show and take a nap."

I took a deep breath. I did not want to do it.

"Fine," I finally said, "I'll do it tomorrow. But I want to get some work done and see a few friends today. I am not ready right now."

I made my appointment and the conversation ended. Then I forced the thought of the MRI into the back of my mind, where I could happily ignore it for a full day.

# # #

On a sunny summer morning in New York City, I walked into a clean, modern office adjacent to a movie theater in midtown Manhattan for my preventive screening MRI. The space had comfortable chairs, art on the walls, and a friendly staff who immediately tried to put my fears to rest. They told me the MRI machine was well lit inside, that I could speak to my radiology tech at any time, and—to prevent me from getting bored—I could listen to piped-in music or watch television while my scan was in progress. The MRI would also take less than an hour. I could do anything for less than an hour . . . right?

Preventive MRIs start at just under $1,000 and can go up to around $5,000. After I paid and reviewed my health history with a nurse, I got dressed in a set of gray scrubs, laid back on a padded table next to the opening of a large, tubular machine. A tech added cages around my head and body, a mirrored virtual reality headset to my eyes, and began to roll me backward. *Here goes nothing,* I said to myself. As the machine powered on, I felt the table move slowly back into the tube.

It was terrible for me. I had to work to steady my breath and not move my body, and I scrunched my eyes as tightly closed as possible. I am *so* claustrophobic. I sang *The Little Mermaid*'s "Part of Your World" on repeat, and it was all I clung to. I sing that song every night to my four babies, and I have since they were born. It's the only calming tactic that works for me in the machine. I knew then and know now that I won't run out of oxygen, but my nerves always get the better of me.

A long hour later, the MRI finally ended and I was rolled back out into the room, where the tech told me a radiologist would review my results. If anything called for immediate attention, someone would call me, and the office would send me an email, which would direct me to download an app to review the results. Great, another app.

I walked outside and set my mind to enjoying the big city. I had great memories in New York, including graduating from NYU's Stern Business School and giving birth to our first two children, our fourteen-year-old twins, Abraham and Ruth. New York City felt like a second home to me, and though I didn't know it yet, the city had just given me another gift: the scan that would transform my future.

A week later, the results were in: The MRI had located my IUD, a minor sinus infection, a few nodules on my thyroid—no doubt the product of the thyroid condition I'd known about and had been treating since my twenties—and a small spot on my lungs.

Indeterminate bandlike pulmonary infiltrates of the right middle lobe measuring approximately 3.8 cm.

The wording to describe the spot was overly medical, but between my pulmonologist dad and my radiologist friend Kim, I knew I'd be able to decipher it. I also reviewed the report with Adam, and we both felt confident nothing was urgent or concerning. At that moment, the findings said my spot was "minor," and with no symptoms, there was little reason for concern. It recommended following up in a few months if I did become symptomatic.

Fine, I can handle that.

The Respiratory System

Let's take a deep breath and start from the beginning. I grew up in Santa Barbara, California, as the oldest of three with both parents practicing medicine. My parents met while my mom was in medical school and my dad was doing his residency, and Mom became a pediatrician while Dad became a pulmonary specialist working in critical care. My brothers ultimately followed their paths into medicine and

(Continued . . .)

are both orthopedic surgeons who practice together every day in Santa Barbara. I took a different route: Even though I studied molecular and cell biology at the University of California, Berkeley, I went into the health-care industry, but on the business side. After a few years of traveling four days a week from coast to coast, I moved into health-care tech in San Francisco, then decided to go to business school in New York. I got married, moved into finance, had four kids, and landed in Nashville a decade later.

Medical procedures and care were daily topics of conversation during my childhood while we were sitting around the dinner table.

"I did a few bronchs today and have another one early tomorrow morning," my dad would say as we settled down at the table after one of his long shifts. Dad didn't have to explain. I knew bronch was a bronchoscopy, a low-risk outpatient procedure used to biopsy masses in the lungs. He did them day in and day out to diagnose all kinds of lung diseases, from cancer to pneumonia to pulmonary fibrosis.

Yet for all the understanding I had about the lungs, I'd never really thought about my own. I mean, I studied biology all through college, so I get the big-picture stuff. I understand what the lungs do and how they take in oxygen and facilitate its transport to my cells. I've also always appreciated that they let me take my six-mile runs and help me at high altitude when I take my kids skiing in the mountains. But my lungs weren't something I necessarily *cared* for, which means I probably took them for granted. Today, I am proud to say that I have one whole lung and a half of the other. I am also thankful every day for all the hard work they are doing as I begin to run and ski again.

But what are they composed of and how do they work?

Your two lungs are part of your respiratory system, the organ system that is responsible for drawing in air, filtering out oxygen, passing it to the cells, and removing carbon dioxide from the body. When it's fully inflated, a lung measures just over ten inches, weighs just over two pounds, and can hold about three soda bottles' worth of air. When it deflates, the lung is only a few inches long and resembles a pinkish-brownish-gray raisin. If every inch of your lungs' surface area was spread over the ground, it would extend to about the size of a tennis court. All that exposed area is what allows your body to process oxygen so quickly and efficiently. In fact, it's estimated that an adult takes in over twenty-thousand breaths a day.

The right lung is larger and fatter than the left and contains three lobes called the upper, middle, and lower lobes. The left lung only has two lobes—the upper and lower—but it also has a cardiac notch where your heart fits, as well as a small extension of the upper lobe called the lingula. The lungs don't fill up the entire thoracic cavity, which is the area enclosed by your ribs, but they take up most of the space, leaving room for the blood vessels,

(Continued . . .)

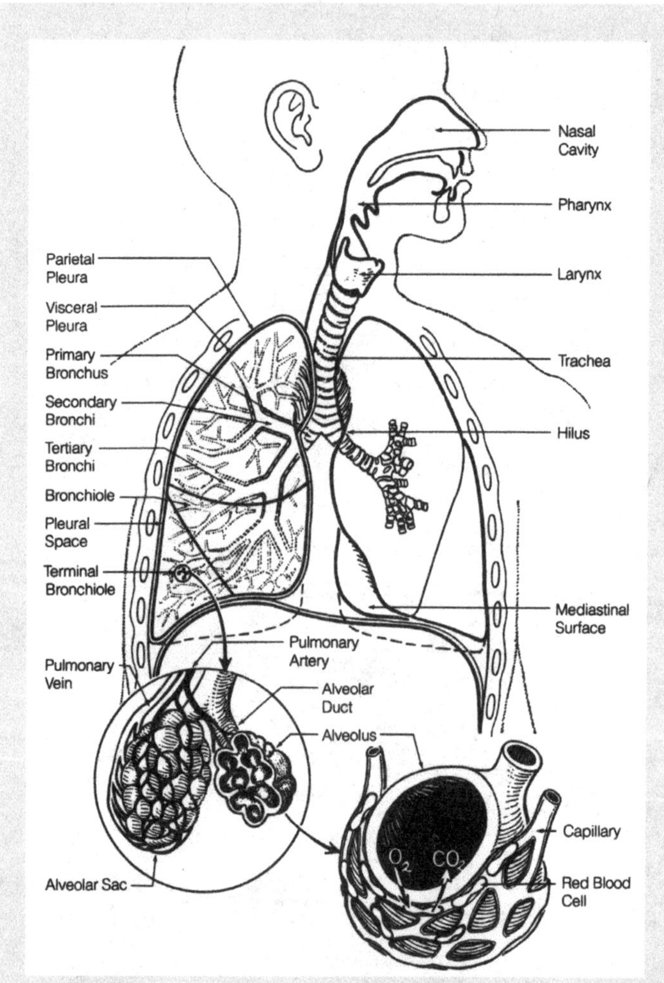

Source: National Cancer Institute.

heart, and lymph nodes that make up most of the respiratory and circulatory systems.

How do the lungs work? When you take air into your nose and mouth, it passes through the back of your throat and into your windpipe (or trachea). As the air travels deeper into your body, it heads into your two bronchial tubes, which then branch into your lungs. Imagine your lungs are an upside-down tree. The trachea is the trunk, while the bronchial tubes are its major limbs. The bronchial tubes enter the soft tissue of the lungs, where they split and narrow into smaller air passages called bronchi, then into even smaller passages called bronchioles. Eventually, they split and get narrower and narrower until they end at the alveoli (or air sacs.) Most adults have between 300 and 500 million alveoli, which are responsible for transferring oxygen into your blood. When the alveoli are fully inflated, they make the lungs look like two large pinkish-gray sponges, capable of carrying so much air that they can float in water.

Chapter Two

The CT Scan

Fall 2025

Not long after my MRI, I called my dad to discuss my results. I wasn't really worried, but I couldn't shake the thought that I had a mysterious spot on my lungs.

Dad was reassuring when he echoed Kim. "An MRI isn't the best tool to detect something in the lungs because they're full of air, so the images you get from an MRI aren't great." Then he went on to explain that I should get an LDCT. Since the early 1990s, doctors had considered LDCTs to be the gold standard in terms of lung imaging.[1] "You should schedule one," he added, "but insurance won't cover it since you don't meet the screening guidelines."

I filed his idea away so I could think about it later. I had so much on my plate, and I wasn't having any symptoms. I was going to be just fine, right?

A few weeks later, I went to my endocrinologist for a routine appointment to check my thyroid and refill my medications. My MRI was on my phone, so I decided to show it to him. Remember, it had shown thyroid nodules in addition to the spot on my lung.

"Well, those nodules are from your Hashimoto's," he said, pointing to the wording describing the findings for my thyroid. Hashimoto's was the autoimmune disease I'd had since my twenties. "They're nothing to worry about, as you probably know."

"Yes," I answered, then I paused before deciding what I wanted to say next. "I know you're not a radiologist and certainly not a lung doctor, but could I show you something?" I zoomed in on the photo of my lungs, with the "spot" circled in red. "See this?"

My endocrinologist leaned toward my phone as I pointed to the circle. "I do," he said. Then he paused for a moment. "Look, I may not be a radiologist, but I know MRIs aren't the best tools for looking at some organs. I'm not worried about you in the slightest because you're not having any symptoms, but if you want, I can schedule you a low-dose CT."

A low-dose CT, I thought. *Just like Dad said.*

What Is a Low-Dose CT Scan?

A CT or CAT scan (shorthand for computerized tomography) was invented in 1971 by a British engineer, and it uses X-rays to create images of thin layers of your body. How thin? The inventor said CT results look like an organ or body part has been "put through a bacon slicer."

A CT scanner resembles an MRI machine, but it's a much smaller device with a donut shaped opening rather than a large, gaping magnetic tube. Just like an MRI, you lie on your back on a table, and the table reverses through the device. The images created by the X-rays are then sent to a computer, which analyzes its cross-sections (or "slices"). CTs take more detailed images than standard X-ray machines, and—lucky for claustrophobic me—they only take a few minutes to do.

To be clear, the downside of a CT scan that you do not get with an MRI is that a CT exposes your body to radiation. However, CTs use very low doses to take images of the lungs because lung tissue is spongy and not very dense. There is less tissue to study on each slice, so you can use less radiation to expose it. These doses are one-fifth the amount of radiation used in standard CTs, which take images of bones and other organs, and research has shown that a LDCT is just as effective as a standard CT in finding lung nodules.[2] Regardless, in a LDCT, the amount of radiation a patient is exposed to is considered relatively harmless.

# # #

When I moved to Nashville in April 2021, I knew next to no one. My children ranged from three to nine years old and had already lived in seven cities in six states, and we were more than ready to slow down. When we landed in Tennessee, Adam and I hoped it would be our last stop and that we'd be able to navigate our children through high school in Nashville. We bought a house, enrolled our four kids in three schools, and set out on a mission to make friends and build a community.

Within four months, I found Kim.

Dr. Kim Sandler is a cardiothoracic radiologist at Vanderbilt University who is trained in the interpretation of chest, cardiovascular, and vascular imaging, X-rays, CTs, and MRIs. Her focus is on early detection of lung cancer with CT screening, and she assumed leadership of Vanderbilt's lung screening program in 2015. Kim's oldest child and mine overlapped at school, and we quickly bonded over our love of sushi, fashion, and medical talk.

Kim's parents and siblings are doctors, just like mine, and over lunch we would review her lung cancer research and discuss the best spots to shop on her next international speaking engagement. Naturally, one day I found myself sharing my MRI results, and though she acknowledged the finding, she also turned up her nose, citing the CT as a better scan for lung specific screening.

This narrative was sounding familiar.

Kim's a fast talker, and she quickly explained her thinking. "An MRI has never been a test that I've recommended for lungs," she said. "I think it has a lot of benefits, but because of how much air there is in the chest and the spatial resolution of MRI, we just don't see images very well."

"Yeah, that's exactly what my dad said," I answered.

"Right. So, what he probably also said is that you shouldn't worry, but if you want to rule out all the bad yet unlikely scenarios you see with lung spots, go get a CT. It's a much better test, and if there's something there, we'll see it. Or maybe we can say that this spot is nothing and that we're done. And, based on my experience, it's probably nothing."

"Am I right that insurance won't pay?" I asked.

"Yes, because you don't meet the screening guidelines. You're not over fifty and you never smoked. But at Vanderbilt, a LDCT costs $400. It used to be $150, and we're trying to get it back to that."

I paused, considering what she'd said. Then I made my decision.

"I'll get scanned," I said. "And I'll show you the results when I have them."

Thursday, September 25, 2025

It was just another Thursday morning. I got the four kids out the door, into the minivan, and off to school. Then I hurried to work, did as much as I could, and drove back to school to grab my middle child for her orthodontic appointment. When that was over, I delivered her once again to school, and just before pickup, I popped in for a LDCT scan booked by my endocrinologist. As I raced out to grab the kids, I requested a CD copy of the CT to shoot over to my dad and, of course, to Kim.

To be honest, I was not nervous one bit about the scan or the results. In fact, it felt good to cross one more thing off my to-do list.

Chapter Three

Diagnosis

Saturday, September 27, 2025

On the last Saturday in September, I was at the Pilgrimage Music and Cultural Festival in Franklin, about twenty miles south of Nashville. My son had joined me, along with some of our close friends from New Orleans, my dad's hometown and where Adam, the kids, and I once lived. Adam was in Kabul, Afghanistan, freeing a hostage who'd been kidnapped by the Taliban. No, I'm not making that up. Adam serves as the Special Envoy for Hostage Response under the US Department of State, so he negotiates the release of hostages held abroad while also running a health-care investment firm.

My friends, son, and I were enjoying the headliner, Kings of Leon, when I glanced at my phone and saw Kim's number come up. It wasn't like Kim to call on a Saturday night.

"What's up?" I asked.

Kim paused. "I read your CT, and, as you saw, the spot is now showing 4.1 centimeters. It was 3.8 before."

"Right," I said. I'd read my results from the recent CT I'd taken, including the radiologist's report. "But the rest of the report said I should come back in three months if I'm symptomatic. I ran yesterday, and I'm completely fine. I had no cough or chest pain or any other symptoms!"

"I agree-ish," Kim answered, "but I don't like this scan. I want you to get a more detailed one, and I've made an appointment for you at Vanderbilt, for Monday morning."

I went quiet. *This is so annoying*, I thought. I mean, I am a big believer in TGIM, and I love a good Monday. The kids go to school, I go for a run, and then I head to work. Now Kim wanted me back at Vanderbilt for another scan. This one would be a 1mm spiral CT, which is far more detailed and gives a clearer view of lung tissue than the 5mm CT I received three days prior.

There went my Monday.

What Kim didn't tell me then—but told me later—was that it wasn't necessarily the *growth* of the mass that concerned her, but instead its very presence. If my spot had been pneumonia or something similar, it would have cleared in the three months since I'd had my MRI. She also didn't reveal that she had already booked a bronchoscopy for Tuesday morning.

"Great," Kim said. "Your appointment is at 10:30 a.m. and I scheduled you with a pulmonologist right after. His name is Dr. Lentz, and his daughter is in your youngest's class."

My stomach sank even further. Monday was in two days. If my spot was harmless, why was I scheduled for a second CT *and* a pulmonologist visit so quickly? And why, again, was Kim calling me on a Saturday night?

"Where is Adam?" Kim asked.

More confusing questions! Adam was halfway across the globe doing important business. He did not even know I'd *had* a CT scan on Thursday.

"Why are you asking about Adam?" I demanded.

Kings of Leon was blasting in the background, but I swear I could hear Kim take a deep breath on the other end of the line. "I asked where Adam was because you need to tell him to come home right away."

Monday, September 29, 2025

Denial can be a powerful coping mechanism when disaster strikes, but honestly, I'm not even sure that's what I was feeling. If I'd been in denial, I would have understood exactly *what* I was forcing out of my mind. In reality, I had no idea what, if anything, was happening with my body. Kim's insistence that I get another scan could be easily explained by the fact that one-millimeter slices are more precise than five-millimeter slices, or perhaps by the fact that second opinions are routine.

What I still couldn't figure out was why Kim had told me to call Adam and ask him to come home. There was absolutely no reason he had to fly back to Nashville so he could watch me have a routine CT, right?

Unless there was actually something wrong.

Despite a mountain of evidence pointing toward bad news, I was still convinced I didn't have anything to worry about. Surely no one with a cancerous mass or dangerous nodule or whatever this thing on my lungs might be could feel as healthy as I did. No one as active as me could ever have a serious illness, could they? Over the weekend, I had shuttled my children from sports games to play dates and still found time to go out with my friends to see live music. Just that morning, I'd woken up before dawn, battled the teenagers out of bed, fed the kids breakfast, and ushered four tired children out the door so they'd make it to school on time. Then I'd turned around and was about to run six very hilly miles with a friend. My head was clear, my heart was full, and I'd never felt better in my life. If there was something going on in my lungs, I was sure it would be no big deal.

Right?

I'd caught Adam on his flight from Kabul to Doha, Qatar, and he agreed to change up his trip as best he could. His new flight would definitely cause him to miss my 10:30 CT scan, but he'd hopefully make it to the pulmonologist's appointment.

"Let's run fast," I said to my friend when we met up. "I have a doctor's appointment this morning." I rolled my eyes, and she nodded her head as we took off.

By 10:15, I was freshly showered and sitting alone in a radiology waiting room at a Vanderbilt University Imaging Center clinic. My name was called, and a technician greeted me and escorted me into the CT scan room. She explained I would be receiving a diagnostic helical CT (or spiral scan) where the X-rays emitted by the machine would travel in a circular path around my body as it passed through the doughnut-shaped opening. These X-rays would penetrate my body at all angles, helping to create 3D images that are far more detailed than traditional low-dose CT images.

The scan was fast. Check it off the list, time to move on. I texted Kim, "Scan done!" and jumped back in my car to drive to the main campus of Vanderbilt Medical Center to meet the pulmonologist.

When I got there, I parked my minivan in the tightly packed garage, walked into Vanderbilt Medical Center, and took an elevator down to the basement. Pulmonology was located there, as was Dr. Robert J. Lentz, who was the same kind of lung specialist as my dad. In Dad's words, "the diagnostic guy." Just as I approached the doors to the office, however, my phone rang. I pulled it out of my purse and saw Kim's name.

"Hi!" I said cheerfully. "I'm about to see Dr. Lentz. What's up?"

"Great," Kim answered, sounding a lot less cheerful than I was. "Where's Adam?"

My words started to catch in my throat. "He just texted me, and he's on his way from the airport. He should be here in ten minutes." I paused as I opened the doors and entered the pulmonology waiting room. "So, did you read my spiral CT?"

"My partner read it," Kim answered curtly.

"Okay . . ." I responded.

"Okay," she answered back, and then she hung up.

What? Kim had never, ever hung up like that. She had never, ever not overly explained everything. She had never, ever had nothing to say . . . until today. Here I was, on a strange journey she'd sent me on, and all I got was "okay."

After I checked in at the front desk and sat down, my thoughts began racing. I couldn't fathom why Kim wouldn't just tell me what the scan said, even if her only comment was "You're fine." The more I thought about it, the more her tone bothered me, too. She was always one to move right past small talk into real conversation, but in this case, she hadn't even given me the regular pleasantries. On top of that, Kim had never once asked me to pinpoint Adam's location. My husband traveled for work all the time, and I was perfectly fine living my life when he was out of town. Kim *knew* that. It just wasn't like her to keep tabs on him or assume I needed him by my side at a routine scan or a silly doctor's appointment.

Or did I?

Within a few minutes, a nurse called my name, then ushered me into Dr. Lentz's office. I sat down, noticed his diplomas, and stared toward the computer that likely held the results of my latest scan. I picked up my phone, scrolled through emails, and bounced my leg awaiting Dr. Lentz. And if I was lucky and traffic wasn't bad, Adam.

Right at that moment, Adam opened the door and walked into the room. He always *just* made it—always in the nick of time. Kim would be happy; he was present and accounted for, just as she had requested.

I kissed him hello and quickly told him that I had spoken to Kim and she did not sound great.

Adam cocked his head. "Who cares what Kim thinks?" he answered. Then, before I could process what he'd just said, Dr. Lentz walked into the exam room. He was bearded, smiling, and looked to be about my age.

"Hi, I'm Dr. Lentz," he said, leaning over to shake my hand, then Adam's. "My daughter is in your youngest's class and Kim Sandler's told me a lot about you. Let me sit down and we can go over your results."

I smiled. "Let's do this." I grabbed my phone, dialed my parents' house, and put them on speakerphone so they could hear the outcome of the scan as well. "I'm calling my parents in California," I said. "Dad's a retired pulmonologist. His name is Dr. Kupperman."

"Hello, Dr. Kupperman," Dr. Lentz said when Dad answered. "It's nice to meet you."

Dad said hello, and I leaned forward to level with Dr. Lentz. "I'm not even sure why Kim asked me to come here. I just ran six miles and feel great."

Dr. Lentz smiled kindly, punched some keys on his computer, then turned the screen toward me so we could look at my scan results at the same time. "Well, the good news is that the spot on your lungs is closer to 2.5 centimeters rather than the 4.1 we measured during your last scan."

I exhaled and nodded for him to continue.

"But the fact that something is still there is concerning. Kim said she's never seen something like this show up on an MRI, then present the same way on a scan. As she said, 'It looks big enough to see on MRI and small enough to cut out. That's what makes it so unusual.' Anyhow, none of us here likes the look of it, and we're going to have to test it further." He paused and looked me in the eyes. "Kim and I both believe that this mass is lung cancer."

My heart stopped beating.

"Oooh . . ." Adam said, turning to me, "*that* Kim. Not my sister Kim."

"Yeah," I answered, "that Kim."

Then, tears started falling from my eyes as the realization that I probably had lung cancer began to sink in.

# # #

According to a 2023 study published in *The Journal of Radiology*, patients who are diagnosed with lung cancer in early stages (cancer still in the lungs and not spread to the lymph nodes or other organs), have a twenty-year survival rate of near 80 percent.[1] Okay, these are good odds. That means that four out of five people with stage I or II lung cancer are 80 percent likely to enjoy at least twenty more birthdays and Thanksgivings, as well as all the graduations, weddings, bar mitzvahs, family dinners, and reunions that fall during the years in between. In twenty years, I'll probably be a grandmother, and there are a million things I'd like to cross off my bucket list before then.

The problem, however, is that only 16 percent of patients with lung cancer fall into this positive range. Am I one of those 16 percent? Am I going to make it to the next birthday and graduation?

Now, contrast this figure to the current average five-year survival rate for lung cancer, which is a dismal

18.6 percent. That means that nearly 82 percent of people diagnosed with lung cancer today won't make it more than a few years. And those years? They'll spend them back and forth from home to the hospital, where they'll undergo surgery, radiation, chemotherapy, immunotherapy, or any of the other available treatments for lung cancer. If their cancer has spread, they might undergo surgery, but the operation won't stop the disease in its tracks. Even with the primary cancer gone, lung cancer is often so aggressive that it's ultimately a killer . . . 82 percent of the time!

I don't say this to scare you, but what in the actual f&%*? Let me tell you, a diagnosis like this sucks. I know I shouldn't have, but when I got home, I ran to my computer to see what my chances of seeing my eight-year-old graduate elementary school looked like. Lung cancer is a tremendously difficult pill to swallow, even if you're one of the lucky 16 percent who catch it early. Like any cancer, it's also a long, multistep process from diagnosis to biopsy to surgery to treatment to remission (I hope). Even if I started treatment right away, I knew I'd never fully be out of the woods. For the rest of my life, lung cancer would feel like it was one step behind (and sometimes in front of) me.

"I want to send you in for a bronchoscopy," Dr. Lentz said as Adam and I sat frozen, our jaws and fists clenched. "We have to determine *exactly* what this is."

"I don't understand," Adam said, sounding insistent. "You said it was lung cancer."

"That's what Kim and I believe," Dr. Lentz answered. "But until we biopsy it and look at it under a microscope, we can't say that definitively. There's a small chance it's a fungal infection. Obviously, that's what we're hoping for."

Great, a fungus! That must be what it is . . . duh. Remember, I just ran six miles!

Dr. Lentz explained that in middle Tennessee, a fungus called histoplasmosis is so common that it's estimated that 90 percent of residents have been exposed to it.[2] Some people who inhale the fungi's spores develop an infection that can cause flu-like symptoms such as coughing, fever, fatigue, and, apparently, spots on the lungs. It was a treatable infection—or, at least, far more treatable than lung cancer.

"Well, then, a bronchoscopy tomorrow it is." I said, sighing. "Where do I . . . ?"

Adam interrupted me. "So, your parents know the news. Now we have to tell the kids."

Heidi Onda, Stage 3A Lung Cancer Survivor, Colorado

Being a lifelong health enthusiast, health educator, and a fitness trainer married to a primary care physician, I was blindsided by my stage 3a inoperable lung cancer diagnosis in October 2018, when I was fifty-five.

The really scary thing about this was that I didn't have any symptoms. I had an ovarian cyst. Actually, I had a history of ovarian cysts throughout my entire adult life, and I knew what having one felt like: a dull throb. Out of the blue one day, I felt a dull ache on my lower left side, and I thought, *Oh, my gosh, I'm too old for this.* My husband's colleague had been my OB/GYN for years, so I texted him. He said, "Well, come in right now. Just come in and I'll do an ultrasound."

He did an ultrasound and found a six-centimeter cyst. It was big but looked totally benign. He didn't want to miss anything, so he ran a CA-125 blood test, which is the tumor marker for ovarian cancer. A normal CA-125 is anywhere between 0 and 35. Mine was a 36. Usually if someone's got ovarian cancer, this is in the hundreds or thousands. But here, everything was kind of borderline, so he said, "You know what, I really am afraid to miss something here." He called gynecologic oncology, and they ordered a CT scan of my chest, abdomen, and pelvis just to rule out ovarian cancer.

(Continued . . .)

What came back in the scan was a mass in the upper left lobe of my lungs and some lymph nodes in the middle of my chest that were also plump. I had a PET scan the next day, and my cells lit up like a Christmas tree. And before I knew it, I was having a biopsy.

I got a phone call from my pulmonologist about two days later telling me that I had inoperable stage 3a lung cancer and no biomarkers to target, so I was basically looking at four to six months of life left and I should get my affairs in order. He said my only option was chemo radiation, and I had a 90 percent chance of the cancer progressing within a few months.

I couldn't believe what I was hearing because I felt great. I'm a fitness trainer. When I got that phone call, I had just finished fifty minutes on a stair climber at level 15, and I never got short of breath. I never coughed. And how on earth could I have lung cancer because I never touched a cigarette in my life. I'm also a vegan!

When I met my oncologist, however, I heard a different story altogether. This guy walks into the room, very chipper, and he says, "Actually, you know, you're a great candidate for this new immunotherapy that was just FDA approved about a month ago." Yes, I would have to go through chemo radiation, but after that, if I didn't progress, I could get these immunotherapy infusions every other week for one year, so just a finite treatment, and it had "curative intent." I asked my oncologist what that meant, and he said, "It means I hope to get a postcard from you in about ten years from some exotic vacation that you're on, telling me that you're having a great time."

I'm sitting here today, seven and a half years later, because research matters. It's likely that cancer would have been caught at stage IV maybe a few months later, when I was having symptoms. And unless that tumor is, for example, blocking an airway, you probably aren't going to have these symptoms. Mine probably would have showed up on a regular X-ray, though. This thing was screaming. It was two and a half centimeters, and it was all jagged-edged and everything.

I went through all my treatments, and I never missed a day of work. I tolerated it well. That's another myth to dispel about chemo. People are really scared. And, you know, there are some that are scary. But this was very tolerable. I never lost my hair. I never had nausea or vomiting.

I'm almost seven and a half years out from diagnosis, and I'm six years out as of January 8th of my last immunotherapy treatment. I'm supposed to be going in once a year for just a chest CT without any contrast, but I have been able to negotiate. I'm at every six months, but because I run a higher risk of developing a second primary cancer due to all the radiation that I keep exposing myself to, the CT is no contrast. If my next scan looks good, I think I'll stretch it out to nine months. There is not yet a lung tumor marker, but there are two for breast

(Continued . . .)

cancer—CA-19-9 and CA-27-9—and there's the ovarian cancer, CA-125, plus CEA, which is a more general one. When I started chemo and my team started checking them, these markers decreased. So, they continue checking my markers every three months as part of my surveillance, and if they start to see a trend in them going up, I'll get scanned sooner.

That story changed a very quiet, introverted woman into a global advocate. Almost two years into this diagnosis, I had never met another patient. There were no support networks or anything like that, and I just couldn't believe it. When the pandemic hit, one of the lung cancer advocacy organizations started online meetups, with twenty or so people and a social worker who would monitor and facilitate it. And we all started to think about Lung Cancer Awareness Month and reaching out to our cancer centers and asking them, "What are you going to do in November?" We were all getting very similar responses, either totally ignored or dismissive responses such as, "Oh, great ideas, you know, we'll get back to you, we've got a lot of time, you know, to work on this." Then we'd never hear back.

I had noticed that the University Cancer Center would light up their iconic building whatever awareness color it was that month. And this happened to be September now, and the building was lit up in red. And I thought, *What is that? I don't even know what that color signifies.* And I read this social media post, and it was about blood cancer. So I reached out, and I said, "Wow, this is amazing, this, you know, campaign you have. I now have blood cancer on my radar. Would you light the building white in November for Lung Cancer Awareness Month?"

The response I got was, "We have white lights in the parking lot that get turned on every night, and doctors wear white coats, and we do more for lung cancer than we do for anything."

I felt humiliated and so disrespected. I snapped right in front of my house and let out a primal scream. My husband came running out of the garage. "What is it?" he asked. And I go, "I just want you to make me a big white ribbon out of wood that I can throw on the front door and at least educate the neighbors and the delivery person that I have lung cancer. I'm not ashamed of it, and we need to talk about it."

During the pandemic, my husband needed an outlet, and he decided to learn how to make wooden patio furniture and stuff. I knew he could do it. He came out of the garage with this big, white wooden ribbon. My daughter made a label for it, and I threw it on the front door. I took a picture of it, and I put it on a social media page that's private for lung cancer patients in Colorado. I also had big white bows tied around my trees and my mailbox, and I took a picture of the scene. And I said, "You know what? We're not powerless. University doesn't want to do

(Continued . . .)

anything. That doesn't mean we can't do anything on our own property. It starts at home."

One picture went viral, and before we knew it, we were mailing these ribbons at our own expense to people across the country. Also, their physicians were interested. Scientists were. Someone told me to start a Twitter account because the science community was there. Oh, boy, are they there. And so I found them, and they were so grateful for the ribbons. They were saying, "Thank you for doing this because we have felt stigmatized by our own colleagues for going into lung because all we're perceived to be doing is managing pain for people."

That's how my husband and I inadvertently started the White Ribbon Project. We're a 501(c)(3) nonprofit. We don't raise money for research. We just need money to construct and ship the ribbons, pretty much. And then we do help with other things. If people need some help with travel to a conference, we do things like that.

Unfortunately, my story didn't end with the cancer.

In August 2024, I woke up in the middle of the night with a tightness in my neck. Then I had this radiating pain in the right side of my jaw and my right arm. I woke up my husband, and he took my blood pressure. Everything seemed fine, but he suggested I go to my primary care physician the next day to be sure. I went in, they did an EKG right away and determined that I had a heart attack—what is termed as a silent heart attack. And before I knew it, I was in an ambulance going across town, I was admitted to the hospital, and they were doing a history. The cardiologist came in and asked how much radiation I had had during my lung cancer treatment. I said I'd had thirty rounds of very high dose radiation to my tumor and to the middle of my chest where those lymph nodes were.

The cardiologist said, "You're going straight to open heart surgery." And I'm sitting there thinking, *How did I get here? I did everything right my entire life, and I end up with freaking lung cancer. Now a heart attack.*

I had one artery that was 95 percent blocked. I was teaching my exercise classes every day, and nothing ever happened. Yet I found myself getting a stent. During the procedure, the surgeon said the blockage didn't look like cholesterol or plaque. It looked like scarring from all the radiation. And she said, "Well, at our institution, if you've had radiation to your chest for breast cancer or lymphoma, and you've had 35 grays of radiation or higher, you automatically get a cardiologist put on your care team, and you're monitored." And I'm lying there thinking, *I have something new to advocate for now, and that's survivorship*. We lung cancer patients have not lived long enough to have long-term radiation effects. Now we are.

There you are. That's my new thing. One of the ways we're going to increase survival rates is to educate patients to advocate for heart care. Or even if it's

(Continued . . .)

not radiation, let's say it's constant targeted therapy, and maybe those things have long-term effects. We hope that we get people on board from all over the country. I put it on the White Ribbon Project social media. I'll send out an email. It's not about that recognition. We just desperately want the awareness out there.

Chapter Four

Lung Cancer

When my dad started practicing medicine in 1981, lung cancer was at its peak. (I guess you could say sardonically that it was good for his business.) These high cancer rates weren't really a surprise. The CDC reported that in 1965, 42.6 percent of the adult population smoked (as opposed to 11.6 percent in 2022), so lung cancer rates followed suit. Many of those adults who smoked in the 1960s and onward developed cancer in the 1980s and 1990s. As smoking rates fell, so did cancer rates.

But—as I'd soon learn from talking to doctors, scientists, advocates, and patients—lung cancer is not a straightforward disease. It is also not reserved for smokers. While smoking greatly increases your risk, it is clearly not the only factor. So, as I sat with my possible diagnosis, my head swimming with a mix of disbelief and terror, I reached back to my college days, where I majored in molecular and cell biology at UC

Berkeley, to try to better understand what was happening to me.

A Look at Lung Cancer

Like other cancers, lung cancer develops when the DNA in previously normal cells mutates, leading the cells to divide uncontrollably. Cells typically have a normal life cycle; they form when other cells divide, spend their lives doing the hard work of powering our bodies as our immune system monitors them, and then they die. The sum total of cells in the body doing exactly the same thing ensures that no population of cells takes over. The opposite happens with cancer. Basically, cell growth runs amok or our immune system fails, and *bam*, cancer!

Lung cancer typically starts in cells that live in the bronchi and bronchioles (the tiny, less-than-one-millimeter passages that branch off the bronchi) or the alveoli (the air sacs that are the terminus of bronchioles), and, like many other cancers, can involve different types of cells. Doctors or scientists can determine the type of affected cells—and therefore the type of lung cancer—by taking cell samples during a bronchoscopy biopsy, then studying their histology, or what they look like under a microscope. My upcoming bronchoscopy would allow the pulmonology team at Vanderbilt to biopsy the mass on my lungs, then study its histology. Once they could determine the type of affected cell, they would know what type of lung cancer I was dealing with—that is, *if* I had lung cancer.

The most common type of lung cancer, making up over 80 percent of cases, is **non-small cell lung cancer (NSCLC).** NSCLC is then further subdivided into different categories, all of which refer to the type of cell the cancer originates from. These subsets include:

- **Adenocarcinoma**: This is the most common type of NSCLC (and what they found in my lungs). An adenocarcinoma starts in the epithelial cells, which line the lungs and create mucus. Epithelial cells also exist in other organs that have glands such as the breasts, ovaries, and colon, and, in fact, adenocarcinoma is the most common type of colorectal cancer because the colon produces mucus. While the majority of people with adenocarcinomas smoke or used to smoke, it's also the most common type of NSCLC developed by nonsmokers, women, and younger people. Today, more nonsmoking women than nonsmoking men are diagnosed with adenocarcinomas each year, a frightening and mysterious trend that I will discuss in detail later in this book.
- **Squamous Cell Carcinoma**: Squamous cells are flat, rough cells that line the inside of the airways leading into the lungs. Squamous cells also help

make up the skin, the bladder, the kidneys, the esophagus, the anus, and other organs throughout the body. Most people diagnosed with squamous cell carcinoma smoke or used to smoke, and the cancer is most often found in the middle of the lung.

- **Large cell (undifferentiated) carcinoma and large cell neuroendocrine carcinoma (LCNEC)**: LCNEC is a subset of large cell carcinoma. Both are fast-growing cancers that can begin anywhere in the lungs.

The other major type of lung cancer is **small cell lung cancer (SCLC),** which grows very quickly and is far less treatable than NSCLC. About 10 to 15 percent of people with lung cancer have SCLC, and it is most often diagnosed after it has already spread to other parts of the body. There are also other, rarer types of cancer including **lung carcinoids, adenoid cystic carcinomas, lymphomas**, and **sarcomas**, all of which occur in less than 5 percent of cases and are treated differently than NSCLC and SCLC.

As I said, I was diagnosed with an adenocarcinoma, the most common type of cancer among never-smoking women. But let's back up again. I had no symptoms. None! Remember, I ran six miles the morning of my scan. Most people actually do not find their lung cancer until they develop symptoms. And then, to be honest, it is too late. I talked to my dad at length about what he experienced as the "diagnostic guy" who was the first line of defense for people experiencing a problem with their lungs, and he responded that most lung cancer patients present with symptoms that can be confused with a lot of other illnesses like emphysema or pneumonia–or even something as simple as a cold. At first, a doctor might think it's one problem, but then they discover it's actually a bigger one: cancer. "Typically, there is a cough, or some shortness of breath later on, maybe coughing up blood," Dad said. "Occasionally chest pain, but that's less likely. And sometimes a nodule or mass just shows up on a chest X-ray that you would do for a different reason. Unfortunately, as lung cancer progresses, these symptoms can worsen, and they often go along with hoarseness, fatigue, weight loss, or bone pain (as the lung cancer spreads into the bones)."

I didn't experience *any* of these symptoms, despite the fact that I had a tumor the size of a walnut sitting in my right lung. The cancer measured an inch or so top to bottom but was not affecting my lung capacity at all. Without that scan I would have likely developed a cough or other symptoms within a few months and brushed it off as a cold or exhaustion related to four kids, work, and a hectic schedule. Tired is just part of being a mom, right? Probably. Or sometimes, not at all. . . .

The question remains: Why did I get lung cancer? Did my lifestyle or hereditary factors put me at risk? I don't know why I got lung cancer, and I may never know, but the following risk factors are what typically lead to the development of the disease.

Risk Factors for Lung Cancer

If I'd walked into my dad's office, or any pulmonologist's office, ten years ago and asked if I was at risk for the disease, he'd say the data didn't support it. And it definitely does not. So, what *are* the factors that put a person more at risk for lung cancer? This is a rapidly evolving question, but I'll try to get to the bottom of it.

Cigarette smoking is by far the greatest risk factor for developing lung cancer, estimated to be the cause of at least 80 percent of NSCLC cases and likely higher for SCLC. In fact, the Centers for Disease Control and Prevention (CDC) reports that people who smoke cigarettes are 15 to 30 percent more likely to get lung cancer than people who have never smoked.[1] Dad was right—you should stay away from cigarettes! Cigarette smoke contains at least seventy known carcinogens, including:

- Acetaldehyde
- Arsenic
- Benzene
- Cadmium

- Formaldehyde
- Hydrazine
- Lead
- Nickel
- Polycyclic aromatic hydrocarbons (PAHs)
- Radioactive elements such as uranium-235
- Polonium-210
- Tobacco-specific nitrosamines (TSNAs)
- Vinyl chloride

If these chemicals aren't eliminated from the body, they can cause cell mutations, and cells with abnormal mutations may divide uncontrollably. That's when the cancer begins to develop.

However, recent studies have shown that former smokers who quit and don't pick up the habit again for ten to fifteen years decrease their likelihood of developing the disease by 50 percent.[2] That's a huge percentage that speaks to how resilient our lungs are. While the risk is still there, this is great news for those who decide to quit smoking. So, I have a word of advice: QUIT NOW!

While the number of people **smoking cigars and pipes** has greatly decreased over the years, it can't be overlooked as a risk factor for developing lung cancer. Cigar and pipe smoke contains many of the same chemicals that cigarette smoke does, including a lot of carcinogens. The same holds true for **secondhand smoke,** and research has found significant levels of tobacco-specific lung carcinogens in the bodies of never smokers who were exposed to it.[3] In fact, it's estimated that people regularly exposed to secondhand smoke increase their risk of developing lung cancer by 20 to 30 percent.[4] More advice: Quit now and ask the people you live with to do the same.

Next up on the list of lifestyle risk factors that contribute to lung cancer is **radon**. Never heard of it? You're not alone. But get this: Radon is estimated to cause 12 percent of lung cancer cases, making it the second leading cause of cancer behind cigarette smoking and the leading cause of cancer in never-smokers. Radon is a radioactive gas emitted when the isotopes present in uranium buried deep beneath the earth break down. While it's harmless when it's released outdoors, levels can build up indoors in closed-in areas such as your basement, or even throughout your house. Many radioactive gases can travel through your bloodstream into various parts of your body, including your bones, but radon stays in your lungs' air sacs, and as it breaks down, it releases radioactivity that can lead to cellular mutations.

Radon exists all over the world. In fact, I grew up in Santa Barbara, California, a town situated next to the Pacific Ocean on a massive bed of uranium-rich bedrock. Did the radon that was in every house I lived in or visited growing up, and in all the schools I attended, cause my cancer? Like I said, who knows? My case is not clear cut, which is the same situation for a lot of lung cancer patients.

Heidi Onda, whose story I featured earlier in this book, told me that when she and her husband became empty nesters, they repurposed their basement from their three children's play space into a home gym. "I ended up being on my elliptical seven days a week for at least an hour," Heidi said. "On the weekends, I'd put on a movie, maybe go for two and a half hours. And then two years later, I have late-stage lung cancer." Heidi's son, who is an environmental engineer, urged her to get the basement tested for radon, and she discovered that the levels were twice what is considered actionable by the Environmental Protection Agency (EPA). "The first thing I thought of was my kids," she said. "The youngest was two and a half when we moved into this house. I can't prove anything. But it sure is suspicious."

Good news—you aren't at the mercy of radon if you get ahead of it. Radon detectors are easy to find and cost anywhere from $75 to $350, and experts recommend that every home have them, whether you live in a radon hot zone or not. Much like carbon monoxide or smoke detectors, radon detectors attach to the wall and keep track of levels. Heidi pointed out that her detector is a continuous monitoring system, so it notifies her through an app if her basement exceeds recommended radon limits, which may happen when soil levels shift from precipitation or other changes over time.

If need be, there are companies that can come in to set up radon mitigation systems in your home. This entails installing a pipe into a hole in your home's foundation, then activating a fan at the top of the pipe that pulls air out of the base of your house. A radon mitigation system can cost a few thousand dollars to install and many states have radon mitigation laws that require home sellers to disclose, test for, or mitigate radon levels before closing.

Exposure to **workplace and home carcinogens** is another risk factor for developing lung cancer. Asbestos, arsenic, beryllium, cadmium, silica, vinyl chloride, nickel compounds, chromium compounds, coal products, mustard gas, and chloromethyl ethers are all chemicals that may kick off the metabolic processes leading to tumor growth. People who work in construction, the textile industry, mining, or any kind of manufacturing may be exposed to some of all these lung cancer–causing agents in the workplace. In addition, cooking fumes contain carcinogens, including aldehydes, heterocyclic amines, polycyclic aromatic hydrocarbons, fat aerosols and particulate matters. All of these chemicals have been linked to lung cancer, so if you cook regularly on your stovetop, be sure to use a fan and keep your cooking space properly ventilated.

Finally, one of the burgeoning areas of lung cancer research concerns the **genetic risk** factors for the disease. Smoking has overwhelmingly dominated the conversation surrounding lung cancer for so long that most of the money and research efforts have been geared toward understanding the connection and lowering smoking rates. This has been key to the overall reduction of lung cancer in the United States. That's the good news! The bad news is that, even as smoking rates have declined, the rate of never-smokers getting lung cancer hasn't gone down as precipitously. This leads researchers to wonder what else is causing the disease. Clearly, there are other risk factors for lung cancer besides lifestyle and environmental ones, and we're just beginning to understand them. Nonetheless, there are a few areas where the link between genetics and lung cancer is clear.

First, if you have a **personal history of cancer**, you're at greater risk of developing other cancers, with lung cancer being the most likely.[5] For example, my mom had breast cancer in her forties, so she's now more likely than others to develop lung cancer. Scientists don't fully understand why this is the case. It could be because of exposure to radiation or chemotherapy during treatment, or it could have to do with the mechanism of the gene mutations involved in the development of cancer, but the mystery underscores the need for more research.

Second, if you have a **family history of lung cancer**, you're at greater risk for the disease even if you've never smoked a cigarette.[6] Once again, scientists don't fully understand if the connection is due to shared environmental exposures or an inherited genetic mutation—or their interaction—but the connection between familial history and your own cancer risk has been firmly established.

Chapter Five

Women and Lung Cancer

Monday, September 29, 2025

Hearing Dr. Lentz's words, I was frozen and could hardly breathe. *Lung cancer? How did this happen?* I stared down, realizing how ridiculous it all sounded. I looked fine, felt fine, and had no symptoms. This must be a mistake. Wrong scan, wrong person. Remember, I just ran six miles. . . .

And the kids, we have to tell the kids! As Adam and I stumbled out of the basement at Vanderbilt, we tried to discuss sharing the news with our four children. Finally, we hatched a plan: I'd go home, make myself look like I hadn't spent the morning sobbing, and try to regroup and act normal. Adam would grab the kids from school and bring them home. Then we'd tell them. We would have to simplify the discussion for the eight-year-old, but we would give enough detail that the twelve-year-old and fourteen-year-old twins would understand the implications.

My thoughts were racing. Would they be upset or ask a million questions? Would the teenagers freeze or pretend this was not actually happening? What if they cried? My heart broke when my kids cried. I started to give myself a little pep talk. I can do this, right? Yes, I can! Then I began to doubt myself. I mean, how was I going to do this, and how was I going to avoid the fear I knew they'd have? How would I avoid showing them *I* was scared?

There were so many issues in front of me, but I was adamant about one thing: We could not and would not use the "C" word.

"Also, no crying," I said to Adam. "And maybe we should keep what we say really science-y so it sounds almost boring. Anything to make lung cancer seem, you know, not like lung cancer."

Adam sighed and headed toward school. It was his turn to battle the carpool line.

I hurried home so I could get situated before the kids walked in. Before I knew it, I heard the door open, and felt my stomach drop down to the floor.

"Hey, Mom," my fourteen-year-old daughter said, putting down her backpack and walking to the refrigerator to get a snack.

"Hi," I answered, trying to sound as cheery as I could be.

Adam walked into the kitchen, followed by our three other kids, who were also on their way to get snacks. "Let's sit down, all of us, together," Adam said, motioning toward the living room.

The kids looked at Adam like he'd just landed a spaceship in the middle of our backyard. He motioned again, this time with more authority, and eventually they marched into the living room one by one. When they'd found their places on the white couch, my oldest daughter piped up.

"You're both being so weird. What's going on? Are you guys getting a divorce?"

Time stopped as I tried to process what she'd asked. "Uhhh. No . . ." I answered. "Why do you say that?"

"Because Dad never picks us up at school," she answered.

I looked toward Adam, and he shrugged.

"So, if you're not getting a divorce, what's going on?" my daughter asked. "Do you have cancer?"

I would have answered, but I couldn't. I had to pick my jaw up off the floor first. Luckily, Adam stepped in for me. "Well, your mother and I weren't going to use that word, but I guess the cat's out of the bag. So, I'm going to be honest. Your mom has something in her lungs, and it might be cancer, or it might be a fungus. But we don't know yet."

I looked at my four children, who I loved more than I ever imagined I could love anything, and I felt tears springing up in my eyes. I immediately blinked them away, knowing I had to be strong.

"Like your dad said, there's a chance it is a fungus," I said. "So, to find out, I'm going to have a bronchoscopy tomorrow. They'll put me under, take a tiny sample of the spot on my lungs, and test it. It's an easy procedure, and Pop Pop used to do them every day."

My kids were silent for a minute, then my son cleared his throat. "So . . . what's the chance that it is cancer and not some fungus, like you said it might be?"

I looked at Adam, and he nodded to indicate he was going to take this one. "The doctor said there's about a ninety percent chance it's lung cancer," he answered.

And before he could say anything else, all my children started laughing.

Tuesday, September 30, 2025

"They were *laughing*," I said to my dad as I headed toward the hospital for my bronchoscopy. "I think they expected Adam to say there was a point one percent chance it was cancer, and then, oops! Wrong answer, Dad."

"They *are* kids," he responded, "and that's a lot to take in."

I paused to think about it. "Yeah, you're right. And laughing did break the tension. Anyhow, after I told them what's happening next, they asked a ton of questions, then picked up their phones and tuned me out, as usual."

Dad and I exchanged a quick "love you," and I jumped off the call. Kim was meeting me and Adam at the hospital, and we were walking into the surgical check-in department. In the twenty-four hours since my world had flipped upside down, Adam, Kim, and my parents had been an incredible source of strength and wisdom, and I was more grateful to them than I'd ever been.

Now it was time for my bronch—the nickname my family had always called the procedure.

Vanderbilt gave me a dorky hospital gown to change into and some even dorkier yellow grippy socks to pull on. After I got dressed, I lay down in a hospital bed and tried to get comfortable while a myriad of different doctors, nurses, interns, residents, and assistants came to my bedside. I kept expecting to blink my eyes and wake up from this awful dream, but every person who came into my room confirmed what was happening: This was no nightmare. I had something on my lungs, and we were going to find out exactly what it was. I was having a bronch, and whatever we discovered was going to dictate my future. With Dad and Mom on speakerphone yet again, we all discussed the procedure and the anesthesia I'd be given, and we made sure to ask all the questions. Dr. Kim sat on my right and Adam sat on my left, and with both of them next to me, I started to feel just the tiniest bit like whatever was going to happen, I was in the best possible hands.

I knew exactly what to expect from the bronchoscopy. Once I was placed under light sedation and on the ventilator, Dr. Lentz would put a flexible tube called a bronchoscope into my mouth, then move it down into my lungs so he could take a sample of the dreaded spot. He would then insert an ultrasound probe through the tube so he could look at my lymph nodes. If any of the nodes looked swollen, he would try to grab a biopsy piece from them as well. The procedure would last just over an hour. Then, Dr. Lentz and his team would analyze the biopsied tissue under a microscope to determine if it was, indeed, lung cancer.

"No cancer, right?" I said to Dr. Lentz when I woke up from the procedure. "You read the wrong scan, right? There is just no way I could run six miles, then go in for a CT that shows cancer. Especially when I'm feeling so good! Not possible."

"Nope, Shira," he answered, shaking his head. "It's still cancer. You are definitely not my normal demographic, but unfortunately, it looks like cancer." Dr. Lentz followed with a hopeful smile. "That's certainly not what I want, and it's not what you want. We've also sent the biopsy to the lab for further analysis. Final results should be in tomorrow."

I closed my eyes, still in denial. Still rooting for fungus. Still definitely *not* cancer.

Wednesday, October 1, 2025

I woke Wednesday morning with a sore throat from the bronch and reached for the Chloraseptic numbing spray I'd put on my bedside table. I gave myself a little squirt and shot up in bed. Back to reality! I had kids to get to school, a library fundraiser at my neighbor's house, and some prep work to complete before the Yom Kippur holiday that commenced that evening. Yom Kippur is the holiest day of atonement in the Jewish calendar, when many Jews fast from sundown to sundown. I have always loved hosting the break fast and was eager to get my house ready for the following day's evening event. We were having fifty people over, cancer or not.

A few hours later, Dr. Lentz called, and I put him on speakerphone so Adam could listen in.

"I'm sorry to say that it *is* cancer," Dr. Lentz said, his voice low. "It's an adenocarcinoma, which is the most common kind of lung cancer, especially for young, never-smoker women like you. The good news is that your lymph nodes appear to be clear."

I closed my eyes as all the blood drained from my face. "I guess you *were* looking at the right scan."

"Unfortunately, yes," Dr. Lentz answered.

"Is it treatable?" Adam asked, ready, as always, to look for solutions and answers. "Because we'll do anything."

"Yes, I believe so," said Dr. Lentz. "I've made you an appointment to come in tomorrow to meet with a surgical team. As you probably know from your dad, I don't do surgeries. A thoracic surgeon does."

"Understood," I answered.

Adam and I asked our last few questions, then we hung up the phone, didn't say a word, and moved close together so we could hold each other tight.

Which Women Are Getting Lung Cancer—and Why?

Beshert is a Yiddish word meaning "destiny" and is often used in reference to soulmates. At a deeper level, however, *beshert* invokes the divine providence of fate. It means that in life, some situations are just meant to be. Like Dr. Kim, for example—how *beshert* is that? I mean, if I hadn't moved to Nashville and sent my son to the same school as hers, I'm not sure I'd be cancer free today.

Kim and I enjoyed dozens of sushi lunches (and still do) opining over her research, discussing her stories and the wild connections between women and lung cancer. Her research (and now mine too) have taught me so much about adenocarcinomas and how they're affecting populations of women today. What I discovered was sobering, and I often wondered if it was *beshert* that put me in a position to be a precise example of how much we still don't understand about why young, never-smoker women are getting lung cancer in record numbers.

Let's see how this plays out.

In 2023, the *Journal of the American Medical Association* reported that, while lung cancer rates went down from 2001 to 2019, the female-to-male ratio of diagnoses went steadily up. This means that more women than men are being diagnosed at a faster rate each and every year.[1] The highest proportion of these cases—like mine—involved women diagnosed with adenocarcinomas.

To give you a snapshot of the scale of the problem, here are statistics from the Lung Cancer Research Foundation (LCRF), an organization that funds research to improve the prevention, diagnosis, and treatment of the disease:

- Worldwide, over six hundred thousand women die of lung cancer each year.
- One in seventeen women will develop lung cancer over their lifetime.
- While lung cancer diagnoses have been leveling off or declining over the years, they are doing so for women at a slower pace than for men.
- Lung cancer kills 1.5 times as many women as breast cancer. That means for every two women you know who have died from breast cancer, three others will have died from lung cancer.

- Twenty percent of lung cancer diagnoses occur in nonsmokers.
- Nonsmokers who develop lung cancer are nearly twice as likely to be women than men.
- In 2025, an estimated 115,970 American women will be diagnosed with lung cancer.
- In 2025, an estimated 60,540 women will die of lung cancer in the United States. It is the #1 cancer killer of women.

Among women, Asian never-smokers who live in the United States are *twice* as likely to develop lung cancer as never-smoker women of other ethnicities. I have no Asian background, but it's estimated that among Asian American women, 80 percent of those who are diagnosed with lung cancer have never smoked.[2] Another study shows that American never-smoker women of Asian descent are getting lung cancer at a faster rate than their smoking male counterparts.[3] Let me repeat that: If you are an Asian American woman who has avoided cigarettes your entire life, you're still more likely to get lung cancer than your brother, father, or grandfather who smoke regularly. That's crazy! Clearly, *something* is going on with Asian women. Why are they affected so disproportionately compared to men and women of different ethnicities? Is there something occurring in their

DNA that can explain why they, more than any other population, are in the midst of this health crisis?

There are a few clues into what the causes might be. The first involves a protein called epidermal growth factor receptor (EGFR), which exists on the surface of some cells and helps regulate cell growth. The DNA in EGFR can mutate, however, causing uncontrollable cell division. This may lead to a cancerous tumor. It's estimated that one in three people with NSCLC have an EGFR mutation[4] (including me). EGFR mutations are also more common in populations of Asian descent, women in general, and never-smokers.[5] [6] A study out of Taiwan even found that Taiwanese never-smokers who have a family history of an EGFR-mutant lung cancer have a significantly higher risk of developing the disease.[7]

About a year before my diagnosis, Kim was invited by the *British Journal of Radiology* to present a paper on the link between women and lung cancer. We chatted about it over our sushi lunch, and while I was fascinated by the work she'd done to dig into the connection between never-smoking and lung cancer, I could still see how much work there is to do. I'll let her explain.

> I went through all of the different high-risk populations: Women with a prior cancer history, women of Asian descent . . . secondhand smoke exposure, all these other things that we've talked about and the

> data that's showing that there's this increased incidence of lung cancer in young women that we do not see in men, and we can't explain it by smoking. Smoking behaviors don't explain the differences.

I asked Kim what *does* explain the differences.

> I think that's kind of the million-dollar question, and I think that there's a lot of different theories. I think it is almost certainly a combination of endogenous and exogenous exposure, so there's some sort of genetic predisposition, and there's a way that women are reacting to environmental exposures perhaps differently. Could it be related to hormones? Could it be related to things that women are doing?

The truth is that we just don't really understand all the causes or risk factors for lung cancer yet, though we're learning more and more every day, thanks to the work of Kim and other lung cancer researchers out there. And as we learn, I think it's important to see how far we've come.

History of Women and Lung Cancer

In 2018, my husband took a job in the federal government. Washington, DC, was not on my list of places I wished to move my family, so we relocated from

California to New Orleans to be close to family, and Adam began making a weekly commute to the capital. I also spent at least a week or so a month in DC with him. Almost immediately, I found great new friends and learned so much more about the US government and the policies that shape it.

One of the women I got to know was Dr. Susan Blumenthal, a physician, public health advocate, and globally recognized expert on women's health. (Again, talk about *beshert*!) In 1993, Susan was appointed to be the country's first Deputy Assistant Secretary of Health and Human Services for Women's Health, and she made it her mission to weave the health concerns of American women into all the agencies of the federal government. What she did over the course of her four years in office was groundbreaking. As Dr. Blumenthal said, "We were able to expose the fact that only thirteen percent of the National Institutes of Health (NIH) budget was spent on women's health. And that studies were not being examined for sex differences. Even rats used in most laboratory experiments were mostly male."

Dr. Blumenthal helped to change this, and in 2022, a full 53 percent of all NIH clinical trial participants were women.[8] But, as she emphasizes, NIH supports only a portion of the clinical trials conducted in America, and despite real progress, there remain significant gaps that must be addressed in funding, understanding, and reporting on sex differences in diseases like lung cancer. Interestingly, Dr. Blumenthal shared with me the US history of smoking. In the early part of the twentieth century, smoking was considered immoral and inappropriate for women. In fact, in 1908, officials in New York City passed a local ordinance that prohibited women from smoking in public places. While the ordinance was vetoed by the mayor within two weeks, the taboo against female smokers stuck.

As the women's liberation movement gained traction in the early part of the twentieth century, however, women wanted change—and some of that change came in the form of smoking cigarettes. Seeing an opportunity, the tobacco companies hired an advertising and public relations pioneer named Edward Bernays to promote smoking among women. He created posters and ad campaigns and hired a group of women to march in the 1929 Easter Parade proudly holding their lit cigarettes. Their walk together down Fifth Avenue was dubbed "Torches of Freedom," as was the movement.

In 1968, Philip Morris created Virginia Slims, the first cigarette specifically designed for women. In 1987, lung cancer surpassed breast cancer as the number one cancer killer of women. Apparently, the Virginia Slims slogan "You've come a long way, baby," has a sad double meaning.

According to Dr. Blumenthal, many of the lung cancer research and prevention programs that were in place when she assumed her office at the US Department of Health and Human Services (HHS) were targeted at men, so the rate of lung cancer in men started to decline while women's rates went up. As women began to be included in the stop-smoking initiatives in the last part of the twentieth century, their lung cancer rate slowed down, but not as much as the men's rate did. Yet few people seemed to notice or made it a priority. The government and health organizations were primarily focused on the link between smoking and lung cancer—and spending tens of millions of dollars on much-needed smoking cessation campaigns—and not devoting enough time, money, and effort to recognize and help the growing population of never-smoking women diagnosed with lung cancer. What happens to a problem when you ignore it? Does it just go away? Nope! Most of the time, it gets worse. Smoking cessation efforts have been vital to saving lives, but only in the last twenty years have people begun to notice that *something* is going on with non-smoking women and lung cancer, and that's why we are where we are now: with questions, incomplete datasets, and a whole lot of women like me getting sick.

What can we do about this? It was a question I'd get to tackle after the surgery to remove my tumor.

Chapter Six
Pre-Op

Thursday, October 2, 2025

It was Yom Kippur, and—lung cancer or not—I was determined that all six of us were going to services.

"Come on!" I yelled up the stairs to my kids. "Let's go! Just remember we have to take a family photo first."

I heard my oldest daughter groan, but within minutes, she and her brother and sisters walked down the stairs and into our foyer dressed in their finest. I was ready, too . . . sort of. My hair was a mess and I was dead on my feet from not sleeping. I'd spent half the night tossing and turning, worried about how my children would cope with my cancer and afraid that whatever treatment I faced would take me far away from them. Adam and I had finally settled into a city we loved with a community that supported us, and now cancer had thrown a wrench into everything. Our kids had seemed so happy at school and with their friends, and now I had lung cancer. *What if surgery doesn't work and the cancer spreads?* I thought. *Who's going to step in and be their mom then?*

We snapped a photo and off we went. Into the minivan toward Temple for Yom Kippur services. After we pulled up and unloaded, I quickly found our community of friends, and without thinking about my next move or how people would react, I blurted out, "I have lung cancer."

There was shock, deep breaths, and lots and lots of questions and worried looks.

"Oh my God, are you okay?"

"What are you doing here? Shouldn't you be in the hospital?"

"But you *look* fine!"

And my personal favorite . . .

"I had no idea you smoked!"

I tried my best to look calm and collected and reassure everyone that I was just fine (mostly). "They caught it early, and I think I'm going to be okay," I said. "Please still come to our house this evening to break fast, and please *do not* judge me here at Temple. My plan is to sit for an hour of services before we head to the hospital for more appointments."

Within a few hours, I was back at Vanderbilt, finding out how the thoracic surgery team would be treating my lung cancer.

# # #

"He's the one of the best surgeons I know," said Kim as she, Adam, and I walked through the hospital doors to meet with my surgeon, Dr. Eric Grogan. "If I had lung surgery, this is who I'd want doing it."

I smiled, more grateful than I'd ever been to have Kim by my side.

About a half hour later, Adam and I found ourselves back in the basement sitting in a small, windowless office with my mom and dad on speakerphone.

"Hello, Shira and Adam," a smiling, mild-mannered fifty-something man with a Kentucky accent said as he walked into the room and extended his hand. "I'm Eric Grogan."

Dr. Grogan sat in his chair and swiveled to face us. Kim had told me that Dr. Grogan had been on the faculty at Vanderbilt since 2008 and was now a full professor of thoracic surgery, medicine, and radiology. Often cardiothoracic surgeons focus on either cardiac or thoracic surgery, and Dr. Grogan falls on the thoracic side, performing lung cancer surgery using surgical and minimally invasive techniques such as robotic surgery. He also holds a position at the VA Hospital, which is just across the street from the Vanderbilt University Medical Center, and he spends most of his time operating on lung cancer patients like me. He isn't "the diagnostic guy" like my dad or Dr. Lentz, but he takes what the diagnostician finds and tries to solve it. Whether he could fix whatever problem *I* had, however, was anyone's guess.

Anyone except Dr. Grogan, apparently.

"This is a fixable problem," he said confidently. "Kim reviewed your scans with me while you were in the bronchoscopy, and we can solve this." Then he turned to Adam. "Shira caught this early, and with lung cancer, we can treat problems that are diagnosed early. I am here wielding the knife, not the poison."

I sat back in my chair and breathed a huge sigh of relief. Kim had promised we were in the right place, and now I believed her.

"I want this out, *now*." I said, more determined than I'd been for the last week to get my life back on track.

"Yes, absolutely," he answered. "We can and will schedule your surgery as soon as possible, but first we need a few more tests. I am a straight shooter with some strict rules and guidelines."

I froze in my chair, afraid for half a second that I was going to have to get into another scary tube. Luckily, not that day. Dr. Grogan told me that I'd be spending the rest of Yom Kippur having blood draws, a pulmonary function test (PFT), and a body plethysmography test. The last two were procedures that would test my lung function and capacity, and Dr. Grogan promised me they would be fast and—best of all—noninvasive. The invasive part would be my lung surgery, and everyone hoped we could schedule that for within a week or so.

I marched out of Dr. Grogan's office and found my way through the basement offices for my tests.

A technician situated me on a chair inside a big, clear box and put a mouthpiece on my face. As I started to breathe in and out, following a series of breathing exercises, a sensor in the mouthpiece and the box began to monitor my lungs' capacity to hold air. The goal was to determine if my lungs were performing at the level they should or if my tumor or any number of other lung issues were disrupting my ability to breathe normally. The test took less than half an hour, and Dr. Grogan received my results immediately.

My results were not normal. They were *extraordinary.*

"You've got some of the healthiest lungs I've ever seen," Dr. Grogan told me after my test, as he was walking me through what surgery would entail. "They're not just good. They're perfect."

"I know!" I answered proudly. "I ran six miles on Monday morning and still can't believe I am sitting in your office today. I guess they look good, except for the cancer," I answered.

"Even *with* your cancer."

As Dr. Grogan smiled reassuringly, I once again felt stumped. On the one hand, I had data telling me I had the world's best lungs. On the other hand, there was a

CT scan (and bronch biopsy) that proved I had cancer. None of it made sense.

"We need to do one more test tomorrow before we can schedule surgery," Dr. Grogan said. "After that, we'll find a spot in the calendar so I can operate."

"Thank you," I said, and I meant it from the bottom of my heart.

"Now go home and hug those kids of yours."

Adam and I raced home, finished setting up our house for our Yom Kippur break fast, and got the kids off their phones and into the living room. Right at sundown, we opened our doors to over fifty of our closest friends, plus a few we'd never met before. We shared my story over and over, listened to advice, reassured everyone that this was "a fixable problem," hugged anyone standing up (or sitting down), and cried more than a few tears. We ate lots of bagels and egg salad and watched the kids jump on the trampoline. It was a beautiful evening and a reminder that no matter what, I was going to be able to get to the other side.

Friday, October 3, 2025

The day after our Yom Kippur break fast, I was due to go back to Vanderbilt, where Kim would meet me and take me to my positive emission tomography, or PET, scan. The test would take less than two hours, was not invasive, and would help determine whether my cancer cells had spread beyond the site of my tumor to other parts of my body. If my cancer had metastasized, my treatment options might change. The PET scan wasn't something optional or meant to help me while I recovered. It was 100 percent necessary to ensure that Dr. Grogan could do surgery and would operate on the right tissue, not missing a single, stray cancer cell that could travel through my body and cause the disease to spread.

There was only one problem: My insurance company denied the scan. Yes, I had lung cancer and was waiting for surgery, and insurance refused to pay for a test my surgeon had said was crucial to my treatment. I'd spent hours the day before—the most important day in the Jewish calendar—not with my children or helping to get my house ready for guests but on the phone begging someone to push the approval through any way they could. Nothing I said helped. Everyone I spoke to said the test requisition was working its way through a mountain of insurance red tape, and I had no choice but to wait till they got the approval and reversed the denial.

"I can't believe I'm in this position," I said to Kim on the phone right before I got in the car to drive to the hospital.

"Do you want to hold off?" she asked.

"Absolutely not!" I answered. "I just asked Dr. Grogan's office to move up my surgery by a week since he's going on vacation and I don't want to wait. I have *cancer*. I feel like the clock is ticking."

"You can pay out of pocket and fight them later," she said. "It stinks, but you wouldn't be the first person."

"That's what I'm going to do," I answered.

I want to get real here. I know how lucky I am that I can afford to pay out of pocket and fight on the back end. I'm also lucky that I have the support of my husband, who will go to the ends of the earth to make things right, bulldozing his way through red tape so I can get the best care possible. Jumping through insurance hoops is a situation thousands of sick people around the country face daily, during times when the last thing they need is extra stress, and I feel that deeply. I don't take any of what I have for granted, and I know I was fortunate to be able to put an essential medical test on my credit card. Kim was right—it stinks, but I am so grateful that I was able to do it.

The doctor who would be analyzing my PET scan results was none other than Kim's dad, Dr. Martin Sandler, a Professor of Radiology and Radiological Sciences at Vanderbilt whose specialty is nuclear medicine. Dr. Sandler is a native of Zimbabwe, and he came to Vanderbilt with his wife (also a professor of radiology) on a fellowship in the late 1970s. In Nashville, he helped build the radiology program to become the world-class destination it is, and along the way he raised Kim and her younger sister. I hadn't met Dr. Sandler before, but Kim assured me I was in the best possible hands.

"He taught me a lot of what I know," Kim said. "I went into radiology because of him and my mom."

As Kim and I began to walk toward the part of the Medical Center where I'd be having my scan, I heard my phone ring in my purse. I didn't recognize the number, but I picked it up, and an unfamiliar voice came on the line. Introductions were made and news was delivered, and it didn't take long before I started to laugh.

"That's great. Thank you so much," I said just before I hung up.

"Who was that?" Kim asked.

"Insurance. They approved the PET scan."

Before the scan began, someone put an IV in my arm and injected me with a radioactive chemical called a radiotracer. While I sat quietly and waited, relaxing as much as possible because the procedure works best when your cells are less active than normal, the radiotracer traveled through my bloodstream. If it reached any fast-growing diseased or cancerous cells, they would absorb the chemical and light up. I waited an hour for my tissues and cells to soak up everything, then a nurse ushered me into another room, where I hoisted myself up onto a table and lay down with my head pointing toward yet another doughnut-shaped scanner. The table backed up into it, and I listened to the scanner clunk, buzz, and rattle for a good half hour, signaling that it was taking pictures of my radioactive body. I knew that any and all of the cancerous cells in my organs or soft tissues were lighting up, and I prayed there weren't many of them. *There can't be*, I thought, *if the cancer was everywhere, I'd feel it, right?*

When my scan was done, Dr. Sandler read the results and shared them with Kim. After they'd both studied the image and data carefully, they walked back into the room to talk to me. As always, I had my dad on the phone, ready to ask all the questions I wouldn't think of or would be too scared to ask.

"Let's go through this carefully," Dr. Sandler said, sitting down across from me.

I nodded my head.

"I want you to know that I don't think the cancer has spread," he continued. "None of your lymph nodes lit up."

I slid off the exam table right onto the floor, curled into a ball, and started crying.

Dr. Sandler smiled. "So, we've established that it hasn't spread, meaning that surgery is the best available treatment option." He paused and lowered his gaze down to where I was on the floor. "Unfortunately, however, your cancer cells lit up. They are very bright. They are *on fire*."

My eyes went wide as I struggled to stand up. "What does that mean?" I asked, sounding the tiniest bit desperate.

"In my experience, that means the cancer cells are dividing very quickly. This is an aggressive, bad cancer, Shira. I'm glad your surgery is scheduled sooner rather than later."

My chest started to heave as tears flooded my eyes again, and I sat down in my chair and started to shake. Then I looked toward Kim, who was standing next to her dad's desk. She'd started crying, too.

"You're going to be okay, Shira," she said, "This is a fixable problem."

I looked down and buried my head in my arms. I felt like a weight was sitting on top of me, and the only thing that would shake it off was me letting my emotions take over. After days of disbelief and denial, the fact that I really, truly had lung cancer was hitting me, and it hit *hard.* This thing in my body wasn't a fungus and it wasn't a mistake on a scan. It was cancer. I had lung cancer.

Suddenly, as emotions swirled inside me and the tears kept raining down, I began to think about *beshert.* I knew I had an aggressive cancer that was on fire in my body and a heart that felt like it was about to break, but something else was happening that was out of my control. There was some safe, protective force out there, and it was purely good. Maybe this room wasn't a place I ever expected to be, and it definitely wasn't a place I wanted to be, but fate had sent me here, and it was meant to be. Between Kim, Dr. Sandler, Dr. Lentz, Dr. Grogan, Adam, and my parents, *beshert* had gifted me the best possible team I could hope for, and it had done it right in the nick of time. Sure, I was scared to death about whatever I had to face during surgery and in the years after, when my cancer hopefully wouldn't come back, but I had good luck, excellent care, and people who loved me. I had four kids at home who I'd do anything to protect, and they would always be there for me. Always. Right then, I forced myself to believe that those people—my family, friends, and medical team—were all I really needed in life.

Chapter Seven
Screening

I couldn't sleep. It was the night after my PET scan, and I tossed and turned for hours, getting up every now and then so I could pace around the house. There was only one thing in my mind, and it was CANCER. I knew I had caught it early, but there were too many what-ifs for me to be able to settle down.

What if the surgery doesn't get all my cancer?

What if it is *in my lymph nodes?*

What if I have to have chemo or radiation?

What if I never wake up from surgery?

Wait, what about Adam?

"If I don't make it, I definitely want you to remarry, but I don't want you to have more kids." I said out loud as soon as Adam was up.

"Why's that?" Adam asked.

"Because I want this new lady to focus on *our* kids!"

Adam laughed, breaking some of the tension in the room. "You're going to beat this. We caught it early."

No matter how much I knew that I'd cheated fate in the most improbable way, it was hard to muzzle the panic that kept rising up in my chest. I'd never been forced to face my own mortality before, and it was terrifying. Whenever the panic dissipated, I reassured myself, *this was a fixable problem.* I wasn't just lucky, I was blessed, and that was because I'd gotten an early scan that found my cancer.

The History of Lung Cancer Screening

According to the American Lung Association, smoking rates fell 73 percent among adults from 1965 to 2022 and 86 percent for youth from 1991 to 2022.[1] That is a huge percentage representing tens of thousands of people who either quit or never took up the habit. In 1965, 42.6 percent of adults smoked, and in 2022, only 11.6 percent of them did. In 1991, 36.4 percent of youth under eighteen smoked, and in 2021, that percentage was down to 3.8 percent. Great, smoking rates are way down. We have moved mountains and changed public opinion to bring the epidemic of cigarette smoking to a close (or close to it), but quitting smoking is not the whole story when it comes to stopping lung cancer.

Screening is one of the most effective ways we have today to reverse lung cancer mortality rates. It won't prevent the disease from occurring but helps us catch lung cancer early enough to make it a "fixable problem" and a treatable disease instead of a killer. Yet, only 16 percent of lung cancer patients catch it in stage I or II, when it's operable like mine. Though it seems so logical, screening has historically been widely underutilized. Why is this? Let's dive into how our screening program in the United States began.

Scientists in the United States began looking closely at screening techniques in 2002, when the Lung Screening Study group (LSS) and the American College of Radiology Imaging Network (ACRIN) joined forces for an initiative called the National Lung Screening Trial (NLST). Using fifty-four thousand randomized individuals, the NLST's goal was to compare chest X-rays and LDCTs to determine effectiveness as a screening tool for lung cancer. At the end of the study, scientists concluded that mortality rates from lung cancer were 20 percent lower in those who were diagnosed via LDCT versus chest X-rays.[2] Low-dose CT scans were catching the cancer earlier and were clearly a more effective tool. The NLST was published in August 2011, and, by 2015, most insurers had decided to cover people aged fifty-five to eighty with a thirty-pack year history of smoking.

What is a pack year? It's a cumulative measurement of how much a person has smoked over time, calculated as the number of packs smoked per day multiplied by the number of years smoked, then rounded up to the nearest whole number. For example, if you smoked a half pack of cigarettes a day for fifteen years, that would be considered eight pack years (0.5 × 15 = 7.5, rounded up to 8).

By 2021, however, a lot of new data about lung cancer screening had been published, including a paper Dr. Kim and Dr. Grogan coauthored, analyzing lung cancer screening guidelines in African American adult smokers.[3] The running theme of this and other studies was that current guidelines were far too conservative. Officials finally took notice and changed the recommendations slightly, expanding them to include people aged fifty to eighty with a twenty-pack-year history who have smoked within the last fifteen years. These are the same guidelines that stand today, and they are clearly still way too conservative.

Why is this? Because the current guidelines cover only the *most* high-risk individuals, they miss too many people who end up getting cancer. What if you're forty-three and have smoked two packs a day since you were sixteen? Too bad. You're not eligible for insurance-paid early screening. Or what if you're a sixty-year-old Asian American woman who doesn't smoke, and your mom died of lung cancer? You might know that your Asian ancestry puts you at higher risk, as does the fact that you have a family history. Sorry, you're still not considered eligible for early screening. Or how about me? No family history of lung cancer, no smoking history, and clearly not eligible—but I have lung cancer!

How Screening Guidelines Are Set

The U.S. Preventive Services Task Force (USPSTF) is a group of sixteen scientists, nurses, and physicians that makes recommendations for preventive health-care services such as cancer screenings. These individuals are nominated for a four-year term by the HHS. Some of USPSTF's recent initiatives include recommendations for screening for syphilis during pregnancy, screening women of reproductive age for intimate partner violence, and checking women over sixty-five for breast cancer.

The USPSTF gives each of their published recommendations grades, from A to C. A grade A recommendation means that there's a high level of scientific evidence behind the Task Force's evaluation and that they believe that insurers and practitioners should follow them, while a B indicates that there's a moderate level of certainty. If a published set of guidelines receives an A or a B, chances are that the Center for Medicare and Medicaid Services (CMS) will make the decision to cover whatever has been recommended, and then private insurers will follow suit. In 2021, for example, the USPSTF gave the very conservative lung cancer screening guidelines a B. In order to help push USPSTF to adjust their guidelines again, there is an arduous process best explained by my surgeon Dr. Eric Grogan:

> You can't just say, "I think we need to screen more people." You have to come up with data, then you have to actually prove the data. You have to prove that you're not going to hurt more people than you're going to help. If we just go out and scan everybody, you're putting them at risk for radiation exposure, which is a low risk, but it does have some risk, and you're going to find all these spots in people—in this part of the country particularly—and people are going to get additional workups and scans. With lung disease, there's going to be cost and risk associated with that because it's not like a mammogram. If you get a mammogram and you have an abnormal finding, they put a needle in you. For the lung, they've got to go down your throat or into your chest and stick a needle into your lung in some way, shape, form, or fashion. If you don't get an answer, then you might end up going to see the surgeon to take it out. That's a surgical procedure for the lung. It has a definable risk.

After the data is collected and analyzed, officials then have to initiate studies to determine the cost effectiveness of a recommendation. Clearly, we can see that there's a cost benefit in screening lifelong smokers who are over fifty. But is that the case for people with a family history, those with EGFR mutations, people in high-risk jobs like mining, or even people who were seemingly at no risk, like me? No one will know for sure until someone initiates a cost effectiveness study.

Dr. Grogan was quick to point out examples of how the current screening guidelines don't meet the needs of people at risk for lung cancer. One of them involved an epidemiologist colleague of his.

> [My colleague] lost both of his parents to lung cancer before he graduated from high school. It's horrible. So, should he be screened for lung cancer? He's fifty-seven years old. He's never smoked. He doesn't meet any criteria for being screened. Both of his parents probably smoked when he was a kid, so he had a young exposure to secondhand smoke. He inhaled their smoke. Logically, you and I would say, yeah, that fits, right?

Barriers and Obstacles to Screening

If the USPSTF expanded their guidelines to include everyone in the world, lung cancer mortality rates would definitely go down. But the key to increasing the number of screenings isn't only making screening widely and readily available but also getting those who are eligible for screening through the door. Right now, only a fraction of people—an estimated 5.8 percent to 18 percent, who meet the USPSTF guidelines—are even getting screened.[4]

Why so low? Getting good health care is a matter of access, affordability, and willingness to seek care. Insurance deductibles and co-pays are often too steep to pay, yet these are often the people who need screening the most. Smoking is a habit more prevalent in lower-income populations, resulting in nearly 17 percent of uninsured people smoking, compared to 8 percent of insured adults. Of American adults living below the poverty line, 19.5 percent smoke, and they have smoked for nearly twice as many years as people making three times their income.[5]

One of the other major barriers to screening is access. According to the CDC, 15 percent of adults who live in rural areas smoke compared to 10 percent of adults living in urban areas. Those individuals also smoke more than others, averaging fifteen cigarettes a day.[6] Yet rural areas are the least likely to have health professionals, hospitals, and easy access to care. Vanderbilt has four imaging facilities in the greater Nashville area, and there are dozens of others not affiliated with Vanderbilt, including the one I went to for my first CT. I can get a lung scan, grab Starbucks, and run a quick errand during my lunch break. If I lived in a rural area, I might have to take time off work and drive an hour both ways just to take care of my health.

A third major barrier for high-risk adults is the stigma associated with smoking. Like skin cancer or type 2 diabetes, lung cancer is often considered a "deserved disease." If you get it, people automatically assume you just didn't have the willpower or wherewithal to quit, and—trust me—they assume this even if you've never smoked a cigarette in your life. Smoking is so unhealthy that the federal government and twenty-eight states ban it in workplaces, restaurants, and bars.[7] People may be so ashamed that they hide their habit from their doctors, fib about the amount of cigarettes they smoke or the length of time they've done it, or—worst of all—don't visit their doctor at all. A friend of mine had a relative who smoked two packs a day for over fifty years, and she held back from seeing her doctor until she developed chronic obstructive pulmonary disease (COPD), which she ultimately died from. She worried that if she told her doctor the truth about her smoking, he'd give her a guilt trip. Qualifying for screening requires a person to reveal and detail their most embarrassing daily practice, perhaps to a total stranger. And as Dr. Grogan said, "You can't get screened if you're not honest."

Lung cancer screening is also the only preventive screening that requires you to go see a primary care physician first. You have to schedule a shared decision-making visit, then get your referral, then schedule your screening. These hoops you have to jump through aren't required for *any* other screening, including colonoscopies, mammograms, and pap smears (all interventions whose development and adoption caused death rates for these cancers to fall dramatically). Mind you, these other preventive tests also don't require you to check off numerous boxes like your pack-year history or date when you quit. If you want a mammogram, all you have to do is say you have breasts and that you're forty. That's it.

Also, what exactly *is* a pack-year? If you can't remember what it is or how to calculate it, you're not alone. Any health decision that requires you to wrap your brain around an unfamiliar term and then do multiplication is more complicated than it needs to be.

Eric Grogan holds an additional post as the Chief Thoracic Surgeon at the Veterans Affairs Medical Center, or VA, and he told me a story about how difficult he finds the notion of a pack year to be.

> We've been trying to figure out, for the last three years, in the VA administrative database—which is one of the best administrative databases around—how many people are actually eligible for lung cancer screening. It is really hard to figure out. We are working hard to use the administrative database in the VA to estimate the individual's pack-year so we can determine all of the veterans who need to be screened. We're developing AI algorithms, natural

> language processing algorithms, and more, doing lots of hard scientific work just to figure out who smokes twenty pack years.

Finally, primary care physicians (PCPs) haven't been great gatekeepers for lung cancer screening. According to a recent study, almost one third of primary care physicians reported that they've never referred their eligible patients for lung scans.[8] Let me repeat that: *never*. Some doctors didn't know about the tests, while others were skeptical of the available data pointing to the usefulness of the test. Whatever the reason, it's clear that PCPs haven't gotten the message about how urgent and vital lung cancer screenings are for millions of people out there.

I know this firsthand. Because of early screening, I was the recipient of a lifesaving treatment I wouldn't have been eligible for if my cancer hadn't been caught so early.

Donnita Butler, Stage IA Lung Cancer Survivor, Virginia

I grew up in rural Maine. I mean, really, rural Maine. We had an outhouse and a hand pump in the kitchen and no shower or toilet. A lot of Maine is an EPA red district for radon, but specifically the region of Maine that I grew up in. We had a dirt cellar, and radon just loves to come straight up through that. So, I had massive, massive radon exposure, which is the second leading cause of lung cancer.

I was born in the mid-50s. The way society was then, smoking was a very normal thing. When I was in high school, they had a smoking lounge. I grew up around that and naturally went into it as a teenager. It's a very difficult addiction. I also grew up in an alcoholic home, with a father who was an alcoholic and a mother who was an adult child of an alcoholic. I naturally had some personality quirks from how I had been raised, and I had a lot of anxiety issues. So, you try to quit smoking when you're full of anxiety, and then you suddenly become a single parent of two boys in the Washington metropolitan area while you're still trying to keep a roof over your head.

I'm making excuses, but the reality is it was a very strong addiction, and it was very difficult under any circumstances, but mine were on the extreme side. I tried many ways, many times over many years. I always say to people, "I don't know of a single smoker that I ever met that wanted to be a smoker, and that's why the stigma hits so hard. We're the dirty little smokers, but we don't want to be." Since my lung cancer diagnosis, I don't even call myself a smoker. I say I have a smoking history because just calling yourself a smoker is stigmatizing.

I was active duty in the Air Force and Navy, and then I was in civil service in the Army and Navy. I retired

(Continued . . .)

in 2017 with thirty-eight years of combined service. Through my work, I once went to a quit smoking class, and there was a facilitator that gave me a line that I held on to. He said, "This is very difficult. And you might not make it this time. But never quit quitting." I held on to that, and I thought, *Okay, I didn't make it this time, but maybe I'll make it next time.* And I kept going until I finally made it in my mid-fifties. It was after far too many years and after far too much damage, but I finally made it.

I retired with federal health benefits. I'm one of the very fortunate people, and I don't take that for granted. I always made a habit of reviewing the benefits brochure, and in 2018 I looked at the different wellness checks and saw that I qualified for a low-dose lung cancer screening CT based upon my smoking history. I did not realize anything more about it at that time, other than that I qualified. I didn't know how few people got it done. I didn't know how few people even knew it existed. I didn't know that it required joint decision-making with your physician.

I had picked my doctor because he was a single-doctor practice, and I had grown up in the era of house calls. I was very comfortable with that simplicity, but it wasn't a good relationship. He was very anxiety-inducing, and I avoided him like the plague. I went to him once when I was getting my cholesterol medicine, though, and I said, "Hey, I want a lung cancer screening."

He tried to talk me out of it, which blew me away. He knew my smoking history, but he told me my insurance wouldn't cover it.

I said, "Well, I know my insurance will cover it because it's in my insurance brochure."

He did not like that. He was a little bit misogynistic. I might say he was a lot misogynistic. I don't think he liked this little pipsqueak challenging him, but I got that screening in 2018. Nothing came back from it.

I had a grandson born in 2018. I had a granddaughter born in 2019. COVID happened. Life was just crazy. And bad on me and bad on my doctor because he never brought it back up, and I never brought it back up. I went five years, and I didn't get another screening. It's supposed to be annual.

I finally decided that I needed to stop having so much anxiety about this doctor, and I needed to go somewhere else where I would be treated with respect. I went to a big box doctor with my list because I always go with a list. Right at the top was that I wanted a lung cancer screening.

No problem, no kickback, no backtalk. I got my low-dose lung cancer screening at the end of August 2023. The same day of the screening, they called me and said, "You must get to a pulmonologist. There's been a nodule found."

By the next week I was in a pulmonologist's office, and he sent me for a PET scan. It lit up. And he said, "I

(Continued . . .)

don't even want to do a biopsy on this thing because it could come back inconclusive, and I don't want to take that risk. I just want it out."

He sent me to a thoracic surgeon, and the thoracic surgeon agreed with the pulmonologist. By the beginning of October, I was in surgery. They expected it was going to be stage I, and it was. It was a 1.8-centimeter nodule, and it was stage 1A, non-small cell lung cancer, adenocarcinoma. Interestingly, no one expects an adenocarcinoma diagnosis from someone with a smoking history. As a matter of fact, when the PET scan came back and said suspected adenocarcinoma, my pulmonologist said, "No, probably squamous cell."

One more stigma, right? Come on, let's get real. I had massive asbestos exposure in the military. I had radon exposure. And I happened to have a smoking history, too.

My understanding is that I lost about 25 percent of my left upper lobe from surgery. But I did not have to have chemo, and I did not have to have radiation, and I did not have to have any other therapies. They didn't do biomarker testing on me because it was stage 1a. If it had been stage 1B, there would have been adjuvant therapy, and there would have been biomarker testing.

I retired from IT, so I already had an analytical mind. I already knew that I needed support. I'm a single person, and I wasn't going to burden my children with all my anxieties.

I was already out there doing research, and I found the White Ribbon Project. I called into their community call. I introduced myself and gave my history. I met one person, then another, and at the beginning of December, I was on the national stage on a patient panel at the American Cancer Society Lung Cancer Roundtable. They had been looking for someone like me that had a smoking history, that had been diagnosed through screening, and that didn't suffer from shame and was willing to talk about it. Because a lot of us won't talk about it, right?

My surgery was the beginning of October, and when I think of it now, I don't know how I pulled it off. But there are a couple great things that came out of that. They are the importance of community, the importance of shedding that shame, and the importance of being able to talk openly. I love my thoracic surgeon. He's an amazing man. Huge charisma and a highly skilled surgeon. But they wouldn't do biomarker testing on me because I was stage 1A and he said it wouldn't change my treatment. I was very unhappy with that because I knew that a lot of oncologists and thoracic surgeons believe that everybody should get biomarker testing. I also knew that in a significant number of states, insurance must cover biomarker testing.

Virginia doesn't happen to be one of them.

Someone in the audience pulled me aside and gave me a direct line to another doctor. I got an appointment

(Continued . . .)

for a week and a half later, and that doctor pulled my tissue from where it was being stored back where I'd had my surgery and submitted my biomarker testing. I learned that I have a genetic mutation called KRAS G12C.

Well, what I found out while I was at that roundtable was that there was a targeted therapy for EGFR mutation and that they had a new trial out for anybody that was EGFR within twelve weeks of resection, which means surgery. I wouldn't be eligible for that. But that knowledge was ammunition when I went back to my thoracic surgeon, not to be mean, but to say to him, "I know you said it wouldn't have changed my treatment, but I learned that if I had been EGFR, it could have changed my treatment." It established a different kind of relationship. We talk at a different level now.

I am one of the very fortunate ones in the KRAS community because KRAS has always been called the undruggable one. They didn't have a targeted therapy for it. Recently, they have created a targeted therapy for my particular mutation. I don't have any evidence of disease right now—my surgery was considered curative—and that targeted therapy for my mutation doesn't come along until you are deep into the disease. I hope to never get to that point, but if I were to recur and progress, the good news for my mutation is that there is a targeted therapy.

That's the good news, which brings me to another place. When I first left surgery and first came out of care before I got involved with the community, I thought, *Wow, aren't I a lucky one. Stage I, right? They cut it out and I'm cured, right?* Well, I quickly learned there's a real chance of recurrence, and I have personally met a couple of people that have recurred, progressed, and passed. That was very sobering, and it created a real mental health issue for me for a while. But it reinforced the importance of community, to keep you in tune with understanding your disease. If you get diagnosed with cancer, you are a changed human. You're changed from that point forward. And especially something like lung cancer, because it has such a high death rate that it's on your shoulder all the time. It's always talking in your ear, telling you, "I'll be back." You can't burden your family members with those fears. You need to have a place where you can talk about those fears, and it can't be to your adult kids, right? Community comes in there.

I'm at every six months for scans. My surgeon had wanted to move me out to a year, and I told him I wasn't comfortable with that. At a conference, I asked oncologists who specialize in KRAS whether there was a higher rate of recurrence, and they said yes. Once again, I advocated for myself, and my doctor said, "Okay." He's still keeping me at every six months.

Whenever I go to Capitol Hill, I talk about the importance of research dollars and that you can't start and stop research dollars. You can't get a project going and then pull the rug out from underneath them and then expect them

(Continued . . .)

to be able to pick back up where they were. Consistency and supporting research are incredibly important, and getting a grip on what's happening. There seems to be a huge number of young women getting diagnosed, especially the female Asian population.

I'm a street advocate, too. I talk to a lot of people on the trails, because I'm a hiker. And I have yet to meet anyone who knows about screening. I tell them, "You don't fit the guidelines, but you might have a mother or an aunt or a cousin who does. Screening saves lives. I'm here as a stage I survivor, seventy years old, and I'm out there hiking the mountains in Shenandoah because of early detection."

What I've learned is that having lung cancer caught early doesn't mean it's simple or emotionally easy. There was a period of time when I had to pull back from the community for a bit, because I was so torn up with fear of recurrence. It's a huge thing for us. The whole coming to grips with the idea of recurrence has been a big change in me personally. But I've learned the importance of asking questions and staying actively engaged in my care and not letting doctors drive the boat. I need to be on top of things, which I never was before. Mental health has become a much more focused thing for me. I'm more focused on gratitude and living each day. I do a lot of breathwork now. I'm so glad that I discovered that breathwork helps with calming anxiety.

When a lot of lung cancer patients with a smoking history meet young people in the late stages of the disease who have no known risk factors, they tend to suffer from even more shame. They want to hide their history. There is a break in the community in that we've got the ones with the smoking history side and then you've got the young lung cancer patients. I try to bridge that by embracing them. We all have our own story. We all bring to this our own story and a united voice, and we need that voice to come together and go forward and fight. We don't all have the same story, but we all have the same disease.

Chapter Eight
Surgery

Monday, October 6

It was surgery day, and I was ready—or so I told myself. At the very least, I'd done everything I could to be mentally prepared.

My first priority had been to make life seem "normal" for my kids.

Over the weekend, we all kept up our regular schedule of soccer games, homework, and Sunday school. I pulled on my sneakers, put my hair into a messy side bun, and drove the white minivan all over Nashville, hustling my children from one place to another. I tried as hard as possible to be the same old mom I'd been for the last fourteen years, but I knew I was kidding myself. I might not have "looked sick," and in a way, I wasn't, but lung cancer had already fundamentally changed me. I'd once thought I was one of those indestructible women who could balance everything—I'd graduated from school *and* had four kids, thank you very much—but cancer had slapped me in the face and made it clear that *it* was in charge.

While I downplayed my cancer to the kids, I didn't keep it a secret from anyone else. I was in the grips of a disease so heavily stigmatized that patients go to their graves believing their illness is their fault, and that felt so wrong. There's no shame in having cancer. People get it for a million different reasons. So, over the weekend, I told my story to as many people as I could, just like I had at our Yom Kippur break fast. When I walked into my synagogue to take my children to Sunday school, there was a women's group meeting, deep in a discussion, and I marched over and sat down with them. When their conversation came to a natural pause, I said hello and told them I had lung cancer and was having surgery to remove it the next day. I said I hadn't smoked—not that it mattered—and that this disease could affect anyone. I urged them to get screened, explained my experience, and told them how hopeful I was about the future. Not just *my* future, but that of anyone even the tiniest bit at risk.

The entire weekend before my surgery, it was almost like I could feel the cancer on fire inside me, and it was pushing me toward something. I was suddenly a part of a club I never expected to be in and didn't want to be in, and now I had to act on it. My first act of service was to talk about my cancer.

Dr. Grogan had explained to me that for people like me with early-stage lung cancer—meaning cancer that's localized and hasn't spread—surgery is the best treatment option. If you can remove the tumor, some of the surrounding lung tissue, and any lymph nodes that may have been affected, you can call yourself cancer free. He said I'd likely have to undergo some form of treatment after my surgery to help prevent a recurrence, but I wouldn't know what that treatment was until my blood and tissues were analyzed in the lab. I'd meet with my oncologist a week or so after surgery, and that doctor would lay it all out then. In the meantime, I needed to pour all my energy into healing from my surgery.

"Is it just you operating in the surgery or will you have students alongside?" I asked.

"And is there anything we can do to ensure Shira gets the best possible care?" Adam added.

Dr. Grogan smiled. "Well, I'll be doing the surgery," he answered, "but as far as the best possible care, that's not up to me. I'm going to treat you like I treat everyone else. My residents close my sutures for me. I don't suture." Dr. Grogan went on to explain that recent studies show that doctor's families and VIP patients often have subpar outcomes since all the extra focus and care spent on them causes mix-ups and mistakes.[1] Instead of making sure patients secure the best possible time for surgery or have a veteran physician stitch them up, a surgical team should spend their time doing what they do best: cutting out the problem.

His explanation made a lot of sense, but Adam and I were still skeptical. These were my lungs he was talking about, and I only have one set of them.

"Oh, no, these twenty-three-year-olds are at the top of their game," he insisted. "Trust me. I also don't recommend you move to a fancy hospital room. You should stay on the ICU floor with the nurses that I trust. The nurses who care for patients like you day in and day out. They're the best."

Fine! As long as I could close the door on what had been the most dramatic week of my life, I'd be happy.

"Okay, let's do this," I said to Adam and Dr. Grogan. "Cut it out! I want to wake up cancer free."

Types of Lung Cancer Surgery

Over the past two decades, science has made tremendous strides in the surgical treatment of early-stage lung cancer. As Dr. Grogan said, "Twenty years ago, honestly, people asked me why I wanted to go into lung cancer surgery if everyone dies. The surgery's terrible, and we don't have any way to screen and find it early, and everybody presents in late-stage disease. And I said, 'That sounds like a lot of opportunity for good research to be able to change the field, right?'"

Good news: Change happened. The advent of robotics, AI, and a ton of new research and innovations have made lung operations less invasive and risky, with shorter recovery times. This has helped save lives and make lung cancer survivors' quality of life far better.

Dr. Grogan explained that when he began focusing on thoracic surgery in the early 2000s, the most common surgical procedure for lung cancer removal was through a very traditional method called a **thoracotomy**. Thoracotomy is surgery in the most classic sense. While a patient is under sedation, a surgeon makes an incision along the rib line, cuts through the muscles and one or more ribs, and—while the ribs and muscles are held open with a metal retractor—removes the affected lobes of the lung. The recovery time from a thoracotomy is around six to eight weeks, and most patients experience significant pain afterward, sometimes for years. The average adult breathes in and out twelve to twenty times a minute, which translates to around twenty thousand times a day. After you've had your chest and muscles pulled apart, breathing hurts, *a lot*. Thankfully the field has advanced and, I didn't have a thoracotomy; my surgery was less invasive.

Both **video-assisted thoracoscopic surgery (VATS)** and **robotic surgery**, which is even less invasive than

VATS, are much more common and preferred. Both involve a surgeon cutting a few holes in a patient's chest, then inserting a camera and special instruments to remove their tumor. While this type of surgery still means a hospital stay of a few days, the side effects are fewer. I can say this firsthand because I had robotic surgery. Instead of opening my entire chest, Dr. Grogan was able to enter my chest cavity between my ribs. My rib and chest pain was much more manageable, and my recovery was much faster.

As recently as 2023, researchers believed that there was insufficient data to say whether thoracotomies or minimally invasive surgeries were more effective, so they concluded that doctors should decide which surgical option would be better for their patients.[2] But in 2024, scientists published a paper with even more data about both types of surgery, and they determined that minimally invasive surgery yields better patient outcomes than thoracotomies, with a shorter recovery time, less pain, and fewer complications—all while delivering the same cancer-removing results.[3] Dr. Grogan said he paid special attention to this paper, and it influenced the direction his surgical career was already heading. He also said that the most important cancer operation is a safe one where all the cancer is removed and the lymph nodes are sampled no matter how invasive the approach. As technology develops, he is optimistic that these tech-assisted surgeries will continue to provide patients even better results with faster recoveries.

Depending on the size and location of a tumor, lung cancer surgery falls into four smaller subcategories. The least invasive—which, like all the others, can be video-assisted, robot-assisted, or a thoracotomy—is a **wedge resection**. During this procedure, doctors remove a small, wedge-shaped portion of the lung that surrounds the tumor. The second less-invasive surgery is a **segmentectomy**, in which one or two of the "segments" that make up the lobe of a lung are taken out, leaving the other portions of the lobe and the rest of both lungs in place. The procedure I was set to have is a **lobectomy**, where Dr. Grogan would take, you guessed it, the lobe my tumor was in. Finally, the most major kind of lung surgery (aside from a lung transplant) is a full removal of the lung, called a **pneumonectomy**. For those of you wondering, yes, you can live a full, happy life with one lung. The body is a remarkable, resilient machine, and people have two lungs for a reason.

Dr. Grogan pointed out that if a tumor is invading other organs such as the ribs or spine, sometimes these also require partial removal. And in advanced cases of lung cancer, immunotherapies can also be added to shrink the tumor in the hopes of decreasing the magnitude of the operation.

I woke up bright and early the morning of Monday, October 6, feeling a strange mix of terror and relief. On the one hand, I knew that as soon as the cancer was out of me, I could move on with my life and find a treatment that would help prevent it from coming back. On the other hand, I couldn't believe I was in this position. Even a doctor had said my lungs were perfect. Less than a week before I'd been carefree, active, and completely unaware that the cells in my lungs had spiraled out of control. My mom was a breast cancer survivor, so I assumed I might have a mastectomy one day. But a lobectomy? No way.

I was up at 4:30 a.m., at the hospital by six, bleary eyed and famished because I wasn't allowed to eat breakfast, but all packed up so I could make Vanderbilt my home for the next few days. I put on my favorite sweatshirt, with She-Ra, Princess of Power, holding up her magic sword and ready to kick some ass. It had always made my kids cringe, but there had never been a time when it felt more right, or—because I was going to beat this cancer—more *me*.

After Adam and I got to the hospital, a nurse ushered us into a small room and handed me a hospital gown, and I slipped it on and got into my bed. I looked over at Adam, and he was already asleep. Fast asleep, sitting upright in the hardback chair with his head tilted at an awkward angle. Dr. Kim sat adjacent with a smirk on her face, and we looked at each other and rolled our eyes.

"Hello, Shira, it's time to prep you," a nurse said as she walked in.

Adam sat up in the chair and grabbed his neck. I glanced at the anesthesiologist and asked for some medication to help keep me calm.

Soon, I was on a stretcher, rolling down the hall toward the operating room as Adam stood beside me. When we reached the doors, he stopped and waved goodbye.

"I'll see you in a little bit," he said.

Make that five or six hours. I knew this day would feel like a lifetime to my family. But for a surgical team doing the hard work of keeping a patient alive, the time would fly by. I looked around the operating room and noticed bright lights and a table full of instruments. Dr. Grogan walked in and waved hello, followed by a few nurses and the anesthesiologist. Someone looked at my IV line, then adjusted it in a way I couldn't see. I started to feel tired, and within seconds, I was out.

# # #

"With this surgery, you put the robotic arms between the ribs into the chest," said Dr. Grogan as we sat in his office a few weeks after my operation. He was describing what happens when he performs robotic lung surgery, and I was so fascinated that I'd completely lost track of the time. "You prep and scrub in just like you do during laparoscopic surgery in the abdomen, except you put the robotic arms between the ribs."

I reflexively put my fingers on one of the scars on my chest, where I knew he and his surgical team had cut five small holes about two inches in diameter between two of my ribs. The robot-assisted surgery allowed Dr. Grogan to separate my ribs without breaking them like in a thoracotomy.

Before they put the robot arms in me, the anesthesiologist intubated me, inserting a breathing tube down into my windpipe and forcing air into my left lung. They then collapsed my right lung, an all-important step because it's impossible to operate on a moving lung that inflates twenty times a minute. For the next three to four hours, I was on a ventilator. The ventilator breathed for me using my left lung only. With my right lung shrunken, flat, and deflated, Dr. Grogan cut out my middle right lung lobe and the lower part of my upper right lung. He then enveloped both parts in a plastic bag to ensure no cancer cells could escape from the tumor site and travel to other parts of my body. I already had one fast-growing tumor; no one—least of all me—wanted another to take root and start dividing uncontrollably in another organ.

My eyes scanned the walls of Dr. Grogan's office until they settled on a smooth, oval rock containing a short phrase. I noticed the words "We do this every day" carved onto it, and I smiled.

"That's what you said when we first met to talk about my surgery."

Dr. Grogan laughed. "I got that during my fellowship. The nurses made me rocks with the phrases that the guy who trained us liked to say. 'We do this every day. No changes.'"

"Well, he was onto something," I said. "It worked for me. So, can you explain how you use the robot that did my surgery?"

"I sure can."

Then I sat back and listened as Dr. Grogan illustrated the incredible way that technology is utilized in lung surgeries like mine.

> You bring the robot in and secure it through the holes we cut between your ribs, then I actually scrub out. And I go over to the corner of the room, and I control the robot [using another large machine]. [I don't use the CT and PET scans as a map] during the surgery. I know the operation I'm planning to do, and so then I just use the robot to separate the lobes or the sections of the lung. So, there's the camera pole. Then there's three arms. Then you have the assistant arm as well, that they can put stuff in. [My human] assistant is at the surgical table, in case they need to suction a little bit or if they need to put another sponge in or something like that for me to use. Then you use the robot. The most dangerous part of the procedure is when we staple the blood

> vessels to the lung. They are very friable and using the robot staplers requires a high level of precision. I mean, I used to do all this with the scopes and the cameras, just like laparoscopic surgery, and then we would staple and do everything in the chest the same way. This is a more advanced tool, and I can see so much better in three dimensions. It is the difference between playing a video game on a TV versus playing on a virtual reality headset! I can be a little bit more precise with it, and I can see a little bit better, and I can have a little bit more control. Where somebody else was controlling the camera, now I control the camera with my foot.

To Dr. Grogan, robotic surgery is just one step in what he hopes will be a series of revolutionary innovations that will help ensure better survival rates. I remembered what Dr. Grogan had said about treatments for lung cancer being twenty years behind treatments for other cancers, and I was grateful he'd had this amazing tool to use on me. The robot makes a surgeon's job easier. The robot is the car, and the surgeon is driving it.

"Let me get this straight," I asked. "The robot's arms are now in my chest cavity. What do you do in order to get the tumor out?"

"That's part of what the robot did," he answered. "It cut out your diseased right middle lobe and the lower portion of your upper lobe. This portion of the lung wasn't diseased, but we had to make sure the margins were clear. Anyhow," he continued, "when you take the lobe of the lung out, you debranch everything, including the blood vessels and the airway. Then you drop [the diseased lobe] into a bag so the cancer's not dragging on the skin, and you actually have to pull it between the ribs, so it separates the ribs a little bit. Then you need to close it up."

"And then you got my lymph nodes?" I asked.

Dr. Grogan nodded his head. "Sort of," he answered. "I don't take out all the lymph nodes. I just sample all the lymph nodes at different stations so that you can get the stage of the cancer."

"Does the body then grow new lymph nodes?"

"No, the other ones will enlarge. You won't grow them back, but the other ones will get larger."

There it was again, I thought, the body working like the miraculous machine it was, with a team of some of the world's best surgeons helping it become its best.

I was so grateful to them because I owed them my life.

Chapter Nine

The Hospital

A little before 1:00 p.m., Adam picked up his things and moved from the sunny spot he had found in the Medical Center's brick courtyard. He had been on calls all morning, trying to get in a day's work while I was lying heavily sedated under three robotic arms. It was time to check in on me, though. I'd been in surgery all morning, and the five to seven hours Dr. Grogan had predicted were coming to an end.

"Well, my wife says it always takes longer," Dr. Grogan had joked, but Adam didn't want to risk it. The kids would be coming out of school soon and were desperate to hear how I was doing.

I woke up in recovery not long after he walked into the postoperative ICU. I was groggy and pumped full of painkillers, partly because of the five silver-dollar-sized holes on the front, side, and back of my right side, but mostly for another reason, and it was a big reason.

Because I was down part of a lung, there was now extra room in what's called the pleural space, which is the area between the lung and the chest wall. Snaking its way into the hole on the back of my body and up inside me nearly to my shoulder, between the back of my right lung and my back rib cage, was a chest tube that drained any blood, liquid, or air from the pleural space. The tube was also there to make it easier for my right lung to reinflate and eventually fill up my rib cage. If it didn't or if the lung deflated, I would have a pneumothorax that would grow in size. More commonly known as a collapsed lung, a pneumothorax leaves an air pocket between the lung and the pleural space.

This horrible chest tube made childbirth seem like a walk in the park. Since my lungs pushed on the tube that was squeezed against my bruised ribs, every breath was agony. It was like my entire right side was being squished in a red-hot vise grip. Dr. Grogan told me I'd have the chest tube in for at least a few days, but within ten minutes of waking up, I wasn't sure I could make it another second.

"I feel like I was in a car wreck," I said, groaning. "It's like something's impaling my right side. I hurt outside *and* inside."

"The surgery was a success, though," said Adam, smiling. "Your cancer is out, and now it's sitting in a lab here being studied."

I gave a weak thumbs-up with my right hand since the tube forced me to lie on my left side. The idea that I was going to have to sleep like that for God only knows how many nights, with a sadistic piece of rubber poking through my body, was torture.

I felt like I had been to battle.

It took me at least an hour before I wanted to move. I wasn't bedridden, so I thought it might make sense for me to try to walk to the bathroom. Adam had stepped out to meet with Dr. Grogan, so my mom—who'd come to town with Dad for my surgery—helped me call a nurse to escort me. She guided me into position so I could stand, and then she and my mom stood beside me as I started to shuffle across the room to the bathroom.

"We'll do this slowly," the nurse said as she held on to my arm.

"Just watch the tube," I answered. "Whatever you do, don't make the tube move." With each step, I felt like my chest was being squeezed, and the soreness radiated from inside my chest across the entire span of my right side. I wasn't sure I could speak another word because the pain was so bad. I walked slowly, being careful not to jostle anything, and then, suddenly, I started to sway. Lights out! My eyes rolled back and my blood pressure dropped, and I fainted. I have no memory of this, but apparently the nurse who was holding my arm caught me, and I slid to the floor rather than falling sideways and hitting my head.

"Code Blue!" she yelled, giving the signal that she needed a team to rush in and help her resuscitate me. For all she knew, I'd had a stroke, heart attack, or was already dead.

I wasn't dead, thank God. I came to lying on the bathroom floor with a team of doctors and nurses surrounding me. As they lifted me up to carry me back to bed, I began to scream.

"It's the tube!" I yelled. "Please don't hit the tube!"

"Let's get you back in the bed," a doctor said, "then we'll do some tests."

When I was back on my left side, the pain was still blinding, but I managed to hold out my hand so a nurse could prick my finger. Another nurse took my arm and checked my blood pressure, and I moaned in agony as pain enveloped every inch of my skin.

"We can give you something to help with that pain," a nurse said. I nodded and started to cry, and a doctor walked in to add a clear liquid to my IV.

After about twenty seconds, a sense of well-being flooded my body, like I'd just stepped into a hot tub with the jets on. Goodbye pain, hello bliss!

"Whatever that was, I want more of it," I said to the nurse. And then I fell asleep.

All About Pulmonary Nodules

Meet my cancer. After it came out of my body, someone on the surgical team snapped a photo of it, then sent the lump off to the lab so it could be analyzed and banked. Now that photo sits on my phone, and I look at it sometimes to remind me that what I went through actually happened. Cancer is surreal. The fact that my cells lost their way and turned against me seems so unnatural, but it's something that will happen to an estimated 40 percent of us. Seeing this lump of cancer is a reality check, and it brings me back to the day when my life completely changed.

Thanks to Kim, my doctors, and all the research and interviews I've done, I know more about pulmonary nodules, tumors, and cancers than I ever thought I would. One of the first things I learned is that pulmonary nodules, as spots or masses on the lung are called when they're first spotted on an MRI or CT scan, are exceedingly common. As Dr. Grogan said, "spots on the lungs are like freckles on the skin," and research shows that there are nodules found on one out of every three CT scans.[1] Very few of those nodules are malignant. In fact, 95 percent of the nodules or masses found on the lungs are benign and noncancerous.[2] Noncancerous pulmonary nodules may originate from benign tumors and fungal infections, illnesses like pneumonia, inflammation, or scarring from an illness or surgery.

(Continued . . .)

I asked Kim to explain a little more about pulmonary nodules and what they look like to radiologists like her, and she said that she studies a mass's opacity first and foremost. A solid nodule looks fully opaque on a scan, while a mass with ground glass opacity (GGO) looks hazy with underlying blood vessels. Kim elaborates:

> When we talk about pulmonary nodules, there are three different kinds. There's a solid pulmonary nodule, a nonsolid, which looks like ground glass, and then a mix of a solid and ground glass component, which is what you had. That's most likely to be cancer. The solid nodules we actually see much more often, but those are the least likely to be cancer. They can often be benign tumors or fungal diseases like histoplasmosis or other infections. The mixed solid and ground glass are what we're really worried about. . . . We're not necessarily looking for a part-solid or nonsolid lesion to grow, but if it's just hanging out and it's not going away, that's when we're really worried. The other thing that tells us that it might be more aggressive is if the solid part is growing. That makes us really worried. Once we see a mix of solid and ground glass and the solid component grows, that's almost an immediate biopsy, because that's very, very suspicious.

On the CT that I had at Vanderbilt, the solid component of my tumor was about a centimeter, but the ground glass portion was bigger. But, as Kim later told me, it wasn't just the mixed opacity of my tumor that made her so concerned, but the fact that it didn't go away months after my initial MRI. An infection may clear on its own, but lung cancer keeps growing.

Aside from my fainting spell and the pain from the chest tube, my three days in the hospital were manageable, even sometimes enjoyable. Friends stopped by with flowers and food, and the nurses and doctors could not have been more supportive. By the morning of day two, I was comfortable enough to get out of bed. That afternoon I walked down the hospital hallway hooked up to the oxygen tank that made sure I got the air I needed. My right lung would never grow back, but its spongy air sacs would eventually fill up the space left behind in my chest cavity and start doing the work that the removed portion of my lungs used to do. If I developed a pneumothorax, it would delay my recovery, but it was treatable. Surgery had been the most intense and invasive part of my journey, and now it was time to recover and do everything I could to make sure that the cancer would never come back.

On Wednesday, doctors finally took out my chest tube. I was elated. The pain started to subside, and later that day I was able to breathe by myself without an oxygen machine. I sometimes erupted into fits of shallow coughing, but the soreness wasn't anything like when I had the chest tube.

By Wednesday evening I got cleared to go home. I was out of there twenty-four hours ahead of schedule. I didn't know when I'd be back to my old self, running, traveling, working, going to soccer games, and doing all the day-to-day activities I'd always taken for granted. But I knew I didn't have to rush. Recovery doesn't have to follow a schedule. I was going home, and that was all that mattered.

Chapter Ten

Rest and Recovery

Friday, October 9, 2025

"How are you doing?" my neighbor yelled from the street as I was walking toward my mailbox to get the mail. It was the day after I came home from the hospital, and while hobbling down the driveway wasn't the easiest thing I'd ever done in my life, I needed the fresh air and familiar routine.

"I'm good-ish," I said. "Minus part of my lung. I am trying to rest, but I am clearly not good at that." I had spent the entire morning lying on my side on my back porch, and after I got the mail, I intended to stay there as long as I needed.

My phone rang, and I glanced down and saw Dr. Grogan's name pop up.

"Hello!" I said, feeling instantly cheery at the sight of his name on my phone. I'd known Dr. Grogan for less than one week, but when someone saves your life, you start to think of them as your good friend and your hero.

"How are you doing?" he asked. "I've been thinking about you."

"I'm okay," I answered, motioning to my neighbor that I'd call her later. "I'm outside walking to the mailbox, and I can't say it feels good, but I'm doing it."

Dr. Grogan laughed. "Well, I won't keep you. As you know, we sent your tumor off to pathology, and I have some good news."

"What's that?" I asked, a big smile spreading across my face.

"You're cancer free. We got it all out. Margins were clear, lymph nodes were clear."

My legs gave out and I collapsed on the pavement. My heart was exploding with gratitude, joy, and relief.

"You got everything? Every cancer cell?"

"All of it. Your margins are clear. Your next step is to see the oncologist to determine what your course of treatment will be, but for now, go back and lie on your couch and let people take care of you."

"Thank you, Dr. Grogan. Thank you, thank you," I gushed. "This is the best news I've heard all year. Probably my whole life."

Dr. Grogan laughed again. "Don't thank me," he said. "I'm going to thank *you*. I have been doing this job most of my adult life, and the whole time, I've been praying for someone like you. I wasn't praying for you to get lung cancer, of course. I don't want anyone to get sick. But I've been praying for someone young and capable, who would find their cancer early. Then I could remove that cancer surgically, and this healthy, cancer-free person could tell the world that it's possible to survive this disease."

"So, basically, you're giving me marching orders to go out and spread the word that lung cancer isn't a death sentence." I answered, realizing that Dr. Grogan had told me to rest *and* become an advocate all in the span of one minute.

"Well . . ." he answered after pausing for a beat. "No pressure. I'm just saying. You give everyone hope. You give me hope."

I realized then that I was lucky enough to be surrounded by so many heroes.

# # #

I didn't take any of what Dr. Grogan had told me on the phone lightly. I knew that his prayers were legitimate and that society needs to see—and celebrate—lung cancer survivors. That's why I've included their stories in this book. I definitely wasn't asking for recognition then and I'm not doing it now, but even from the comfort of my back porch, I realized what a big responsibility I'd been offered. I was living proof that treating lung cancer early can be a simple, effective process, and that it saves lives.

Yet today, only 28.1 percent of lung cancers are caught early, when the cancer hasn't spread and can be treated surgically.[1] The vast majority of cancers are detected in the later stages, which means doctors only operate on 20.7 percent of diagnosed lung tumors. The five-year survival rate with an early diagnosis is 65 percent, and with a later stage, it's 10 percent. Clearly, we aren't capturing all the people who are eligible, nor are we screening enough. With more screening comes more early detection, and with more early detection, more cancers are caught in time. More people survive, and more kids grow up with their parents.

My head was swimming as I thought about all the work that needed to be done, and I was itching to get started. But my body had other plans for me first.

What Is Pathology?

When Dr. Grogan and his team removed my tumor, they took my entire right middle lobe, as well as a portion of the lobe directly above it. That upper lobe was what held the margins, or the outer edges of the affected tissue. They then sent my tumor and the surrounding tissue to a lab for a pathologist to analyze it.

Pathology is the study of disease, and pathologists are the doctors that do the studying. Like other physicians, pathologists go to medical school, followed by a residency and fellowship. After that, they become certified by the American Board of Pathology, or ABP. Pathologists don't spend their days meeting with patients, but they often serve as a sort of "doctor's doctor," helping them understand the biological processes and factors that contribute to the development of a disease like cancer. Pathologists spend most of their time in a lab analyzing tissues, cells, and fluids that have been removed from a patient's body, and they look for everything from a sample's makeup to its immunological markers to its DNA. A pathologist studied my biopsy results, and according to Dr. Grogan, they were now studying my cancer with the intention of giving my oncologist a road map for how to treat me (whether I would receive chemotherapy, radiation, immunotherapy, or another form or treatment in addition to my surgery).

I later learned what the pathologist did with my cancerous mass, and it was fascinating. After the tissue landed in the lab, the pathologist covered the margins with ink so that they'd stand out from the surrounding tissue. Then they looked at the margins under a microscope, studying them to see how far the cancerous cells had spread. A positive margin means that cancer cells are present beyond the tumor. Lucky for me, Dr. Grogan had removed tissue beyond the margins, meaning no cancer was left behind. Yay, cancer free!

I don't like to sit still, and that's an understatement. Adam and I moved seven times in less than ten years, and I gave birth to four kids and worked full time during that whole stretch. Did I mention that one of those moves was cross-country, from New York City to San Diego, when I was on a three-month maternity leave with my twins? We actually moved on my due date, when the twins were just four weeks old.

That's me, too much energy. Hummingbird energy, I have been told. But then, *boom*, cancer. My energy was sure to run out.

About a day into lying on the couch, I developed nerve pain in my right side. I'd been told this was perfectly normal; when Dr. Grogan had cut into my chest cavity, he'd denervated some of the musculature in my chest, which meant that he'd cut through and moved around the nerves. Not only did this cause a soft, sensitive bulge, like a scar, but it also caused searing pain across my chest. If you've ever suffered from nerve pain, you'll know what I'm talking about. At its worst, the sensation is what I imagine it would feel like to be electrocuted or dropped into the nuclear reactor at Chernobyl. At its best, it's like being stung by twenty really angry bees all at once. Nerve pain is not for the faint of heart. In fact, if it had gone on for more than the two weeks it did, I probably would have lost my mind.

My right side was also swollen, but that would go down. I was tired, but I had the back porch couch for that. My cough improved every day and the pain in my chest came and went, but it was the nerve pain that really got me. If I could recover from that, I was sure I could get back to my normal.

Then I broke out in a full-body rash.

The pulmonology and surgical teams scheduled follow-up appointments for me in the week after my surgery. Dr. Grogan checked my incisions to make sure they were healing, I got a chest X-ray to determine how my lungs looked inside my chest, and my primary care physician ordered a battery of tests to make sure my body systems were returning to their baseline levels. My incisions were fine, but my blood pressure was higher than it had ever been, my kidney values were skewed, and my liver enzymes were through the roof. I've been on the same thyroid medications for years, yet my thyroid values looked like I'd never taken a single pill, ever. Most dramatic of all, my chest X-ray revealed that my right lung wasn't reinflating, so it risked becoming fully collapsed. A pneumothorax would land me back in the hospital immediately, and I did not want that, nor another chest tube.

Then there was my rash. My itchy, red, unsightly, mysterious full-body rash. I didn't think it was a side effect of surgery, but I knew there was no way I could get on with my life if I looked like a tomato. So, I scheduled an appointment with a dermatologist.

"Have you had a recent sweating episode?" she asked me.

I stared at her, unblinking.

"No, I don't think so," I finally said. "But . . . what does that mean?"

"Have you had a sudden burst of sweating?" she clarified, not really clarifying anything at all.

I started to laugh at how crazy that sounded. "Uh, no. I haven't been exercising. I have lung cancer."

Now it was the dermatologist's turn to stare at me. "Wait, what?" she asked.

"Yes, I have lung cancer and just had surgery. They removed half of my right lung."

She looked at me sympathetically. "Ohhh, I am so sorry. You have been dealing with a lot, and the last thing you need is this rash. So, let's get to the bottom of this. Did anything happen during your surgery that was abnormal? Or afterward?"

I paused to think. "Well," I started, "I did faint kind of dramatically the afternoon of surgery. The doctors initially thought it might be something very serious, but it turned out it was just a typical vasovagal fainting episode. You know, your heart rate and blood pressure drop and down you go."

"That's it!" she exclaimed. "A lot of times when people faint, they sweat profusely all of a sudden. Your body may have a reaction to this large amount of sweat and develop a rash. I feel strongly that's what this is."

Clearly, a week after surgery, my body was still reeling and in a state of shock, and rest alone wasn't going to get it back where it should be. I felt like I was recovering, but big parts of me weren't. So, my PCP put me on blood pressure medication to give my circulatory system some relief, and the dermatologist gave me hydrocortisone. The hospital had sent me home with a plastic device called an incentive spirometer that I used to practice breathing and holding air in my lungs, and breathed with it as much as I was able to every hour. I was determined to take that six-mile run again. (Spoiler alert: My lungs finally felt ready about three months after my surgery.) I got continual blood work for my thyroid, and it finally stabilized around the same time I was ready to run again.

Recovery takes time. I'm not telling you all of this to scare you from seeing your doctor and especially not from getting surgery. If you can get your lungs screened, I think you should take a cue from me and do that as well. Screening, surgery, and regular doctor visits can save your life. They saved my life. I simply want to stress that a lobectomy like I had is major surgery, and doctors estimate that it takes a few months until your body fully heals. Even after that, some things may never feel exactly the same. I thought I was in model health—and maybe, on the surface, I was—but one thing leads to another in your body, and it takes time to regain balance after a trauma. Lung cancer and the removal of a lobe is a really massive trauma. I mean, they removed a portion of a major organ!

The surgery and treatment of my lung cancer put a lot of stress on my body, and that was a body that caught the cancer early and was in great health. I can't even imagine what the stress would look like if it was a later-stage cancer. Lung cancer is the deadliest cancer in the country. It is *hard* to recover fully after surgery, radiation, chemotherapy, when you're taking immunosuppressing drugs, or if you lose a lung or have a lung transplant. Everything is easier when you catch cancer early, and this makes the necessity of early screening even more important, even more crucial.

Chapter Eleven

Biomarker and Blood Testing

Just before my fortieth birthday in 2021, my husband was at it again. He was looking into genome sequencing and health screening to make sure we had all of our bases covered. Knowing that my mother was a breast cancer survivor had always left me wanting to understand more about our genetics, so Adam and I decided to have our full genomes sequenced. I went an extra step and opted for further genetic testing to determine if I had a hereditary predisposition for the disease. I knew that mutations in some of your genes can greatly increase your chances of developing certain cancers, and I wanted to understand what red flags might be lying in my DNA, and what I might be able to do about them. If a test discovered a mutation in my BRCA genes, for example, it meant I was statistically likely to develop breast or ovarian cancer, so I could start considering getting mammograms earlier and more often or even have a preventive mastectomy.

Let's look a little closer at the BRCA genes so you can get a full picture of what I'm talking about.

BRCA-1 and BRCA-2 are two genes that work together to repair DNA and prevent the growth of cancerous cells. Since the 1990s, scientists have understood that certain mutations of these genes can prevent them from doing their jobs effectively or efficiently, which means that cell division may go unchecked. With more and more damaged cells dividing, a person may develop either breast or ovarian cancer or both. These mutations can be passed down through the generations, so if one person has the mutation and doesn't develop cancer, their descendants still might.

The implications are huge: People with BRCA-1 or BRCA-2 mutations have a 45 to 85 percent likelihood of developing breast cancer during their lifetimes, along with a 10 percent to 46 percent risk for developing ovarian cancer. Men with these mutations are also at a higher risk for breast, pancreatic, or prostate cancer at younger ages.[1] I was one of the lucky ones: My results were negative. This means I don't have the BRCA mutation.

Does the same kind of genetic testing exist for lung cancer? Or rather, are there tests that a person without the disease can take to find out what their chances of developing it are? Are there even blood tests that can find other cancers so that you don't have to have colonoscopies, mammograms, LDCTs, or any of the other screening tests that are often time consuming, invasive, and can't be done at home?

The answer is yes, kind of, but biomarker testing makes up a bold new frontier when it comes to lung cancer. As Dr. Grogan told me, lung cancer research is about twenty years behind other cancers, likely due to the fact that it was thought of as a "deserved disease" because of its tie to smoking. Clearly, this is not the case any longer. Researchers, scientists, doctors, advocates, experts, and patients are currently working to harness the many innovations that have revolutionized screening and care for other cancers.

Before I introduce you to some of the innovators I've met on my cancer journey, let me dive into the world of biomarker testing.

What Are Biomarkers?

Biomarkers are physical clues that doctors look for in blood, saliva, urine, stool, or tumor tissue to help pinpoint genetic risk factors for a disease. They also help determine the presence of a disease, how it's growing, how it can be treated, and whether the treatment plan currently being used is working. Biomarkers can include proteins, RNA, DNA, or other molecules like glucose, and they

(Continued . . .)

function like breadcrumbs left behind, helping to guide a path forward.

When a lung cancer researcher or medical professional looks at a biomarker in a tumor, they typically study the tissue's DNA and molecular makeup, analyzing it for any genetic mutations or expressions of certain proteins. When they analyze blood, sometimes called a "liquid biopsy," they search for any RNA fragments or proteins that are free floating in the blood. Unfortunately, these "loose" biomarkers indicate potential metastasis, meaning a cancer has spread so much that its RNA pieces are floating freely in the bloodstream. (For reference, 90 percent of cancer deaths are due to metastasis.)[2]

Biomarkers often reveal particular genetic mutations. The three most prominent ones that point to lung cancer are mutations within the ALK, PL1, and EGFR genes. The presence of any of these mutations may direct which treatments a lung cancer patient undergoes. For example, immunotherapy is particularly good at suppressing PDL1 mutations, while other mutations may respond favorably to other treatments.

Germline (Genetic) Testing

Germline testing is a type of DNA testing that looks at the genetic mutations you've inherited from each of your parents' genetic code. These mutations have been present in your body since you were a tiny bundle of cells, and they've followed you through pregnancy, birth, and beyond. Most germline testing is done via cheek swab, spit sampling, or a blood draw.

Germline testing can be a helpful tool to track risks for specific diseases. Many people choose to have germline testing when they become pregnant or before they become pregnant to understand the inherited conditions their children face, and others—like me—choose to have it because someone in their family has or had a disease that may have a heritable risk.

Though we know a ton about breast cancer and the BRCA genes, we are still learning more about lung cancer markers. That being said, we understand that there are certain genetic mutations that may occur in the germline and put you more at risk for lung cancer. The most notable of these is the EGFR, or epidermal growth factor receptor mutation. Lucky me, that is the mutation the pathologists found in my tumor. (Precisely, I actually tested positive for an "EGFR exon 20 insertion." Say that three times without taking a breath.) Researchers have determined that while EGFR mutations are rare, about 31 percent of never-smokers who get lung cancer have them.[3] That includes me.

Unfortunately, I may never know whether I inherited this mutation from my parents or whether it's something that just happened over the course of my life, due to aging, illness, or an environmental exposure. There's currently a research trial called The INHERIT study led by scientists at the Dana-Farber Cancer Institute, and it demonstrates why it can be tough to pinpoint inherited biomarkers. INHERIT is looking at lung cancer patients who carry a particular EGFR mutation called T790M, and a recent report determined that while 55 percent of the people in the study who had the T790M mutation developed lung cancer by age sixty,[4] most of their cancers were linked to somatic, or non-inherited cells. In short, an EGFR mutation, like many others, can happen independently after conception, based on nothing inherited from your parents.

The other genetic mutations that may put you more at risk for developing lung cancer are associated with the KRAS, TP53, ALK, BRAF, MET, ROS1, and NTRK genes. I won't go into those here, but if you ever undergo genetic testing and discover those mutations, just know that you may be more at risk for lung cancer because of them. But whether they're inherited mutations or something that you developed after birth can't be determined without additional testing.

What should a person do if they discover they have a genetic mutation that puts them more at risk for lung cancer? I don't have an easy answer for that. Insurance doesn't cover screening for people with a family history of lung cancer, whether you have certain mutations or not. Unlike breast cancer, it's also hard to take measures to prevent the development of lung cancer. Many who discover they have a BRCA mutation choose to get prophylactic mastectomies, but if you test positive for EGFR, you can't exactly get your lungs removed.

As time passes, however, and our understanding of the disease grows, preventive screening tests, and non-surgical treatments may become available—or at least we can hope. Genetic testing is always an interesting way to learn more about your body, but it still has its limitations and is anything but a crystal ball. Nonetheless, it may help point you toward extra screenings or taking preventive measures like quitting smoking—or, better yet, not starting it at all.

Somatic Testing and MASLAB

Somatic testing is also a form of genetic testing, but it looks for spontaneous mutations that happen after conception rather than those that are inherited. Germline mutations happen in every cell in your body, while somatic mutations are present in tissues or tumors, and they're typically found during a biopsy or surgery.

The results you discover during somatic testing can be hugely helpful in determining the course of treatment you might take after surgery, or they might not. For example, my oncologist told me a few weeks after my surgery that I have an EGFR exon 20 insertion, but the currently available targeted therapies that can suppress or stop this mutation aren't great. So, my course of treatment will follow another path–something I'll discuss more in the next chapter.

I talked a lot about somatic testing with Dr. Grogan about a month after my surgery. I found myself in his lab giving a follow-up blood draw, a liquid biopsy, and chatting about how challenging it was to find effective blood-based biomarker tests to diagnose and treat lung cancer.

"Maybe four years ago," he told me. "My mom got sick, so her doctors did a CAT scan and ultrasound. They discovered she had lung, liver, and spleen masses, and they tested her blood for liver cancer, lymphoma, and ovarian cancer. These tests pointed to lymphoma. She started treatment for that, which actually cured her of lymphoma. Doctors didn't send off anything for the lung mass. So here I am, a lung cancer researcher, and I've got no blood test for my mom."

Let's take another look at how the lack of lung cancer blood testing compares to other cancers, including its implications. Today, insurance will pay for any woman over forty in America to have a mammogram every one to two years. In fact, it's hard for that same woman to walk out of her annual physical without her primary care doctor handing her a referral and pushing her to schedule her mammogram. (Ladies, you know what I'm saying. It's next to impossible to skip your mammogram unless you want a *massive* guilt trip.) Pretend this woman's radiologist then finds a calcification or mass in her breasts. She'll go back to the clinic to get an ultrasound and/or MRI, and if those findings confirm what the mammogram has already indicated, her doctor will stick a needle into her breast to biopsy a sample of the mass's tissue. This same doctor may then order up blood tests that look at the proteins in the woman's blood because these tests can help stage a cancer, point to a treatment, and indicate that there's a recurrence of a previous cancer. Blood testing is an important *and extremely easy* part of the patient's diagnostic and treatment plan.

Still not convinced? Let's look at prostate cancer. If a doctor suspects a patient has prostate cancer, they may order a blood test that looks at their prostate-specific antigens (PSA), which are proteins made by the prostate gland. Elevated PSA levels can be symptomatic of prostate cancer, and they will help the doctor determine how at risk you are for the disease.

It's important to note that blood tests (like the ones I describe for prostate and breast cancers) aren't the last word when it comes to diagnosing these types of cancer. You can't definitively determine the presence of cancer without looking at cells under a microscope, and that requires you to biopsy a suspected mass. But if there had been a blood test I could have taken just after my suspicious MRI (meaning the one I had in New York City), I most certainly would *not* have waited three months for a follow-up CT. I would have given all the blood in the world to find out what was going on with me.

Currently, there is no FDA-approved blood-based biomarker testing for lung cancer. To get even close to a real diagnosis, you have to take a day off work, go under sedation, and have a bronchoscope inserted into your mouth, through your windpipe, and down into your lungs. If you're me, you'll carry a bottle of medicated throat spray around with you for a full day after your bronchoscopy because your throat feels raw, irritated, and scratchy. A bronchoscopy may be a routine diagnostic procedure, but it's not without risks or without pain, yet it's the only way you can determine if all signs point to lung cancer.

Today, Dr. Grogan is part of a Vanderbilt team that is doing their best to bring lung cancer biomarker testing in line with other cancers. Though Dr. Grogan's primary job is as a general thoracic surgeon, he has an important second job that he jokes he does on nights and weekends. Along with a team of scientists and researchers across several disciplines, he helps colead the MASLAB, a multidisciplinary lung cancer research program. The lung cancer research program and laboratories were founded twenty-five years ago by David Carbone, an internationally known lung oncology expert who now works at Ohio State. When Dr. Carbone left Vanderbilt, the lab was taken over by Dr. Grogan's mentor, the late Dr. Pierre Massion, an expert on early detection and prevention strategies for lung cancer. Dr. Massion built the lab into what it is today: a multidisciplinary center that pulls together pulmonologists, biostatisticians, engineers, radiologists, surgeons, oncologists, and laboratory scientists all focused on collecting and analyzing biospecimens that will further innovate how we screen for and diagnose lung cancer. After his untimely passing, the team affectionately named the lung cancer research lab after him.

Situated on the second floor of the Vanderbilt-Ingram Cancer Center, MASLAB is a clean, welcoming space that, at first glance, looks like any old high school biology classroom. I worked in a lab in college, and I recognized the pipettes I used to use to complete assays, the test tubes used to collect blood samples, and multiple freezers kept at –80 degrees Celsius, where blood and tumor specimens are stored. On the surface, the lab looks so ordinary that you might not notice the groundbreaking research going on there. For example, MASLAB's research findings have already helped lead the USPSTF to broaden the screening guidelines for lung cancer—a monumental achievement that has no doubt saved countless lives.

"About ten years ago," Dr. Grogan said, "My close colleague, Melinda Aldrich, PhD, and our team started a project within a cohort of primarily Black Americans. The hypothesis was that Black Americans tend to have a pattern of smoking, as well as different exposures, that put them at higher risk for lung cancer than other races." Drs. Aldrich, Grogan, Sandler (as in Dr. Kim), and their co-authors decided to look at data from over forty-eight thousand study participants, and they discovered that only 17 percent of the Black American smokers in the cohort were eligible for lung LDCT screening, while 31 percent of the Caucasian smokers were eligible.[5] This huge disparity existed even within the population of *lung cancer* patients in the cohort. Fifty-six percent of Caucasian smoking lung cancer patients were considered eligible for insurance-paid LDCT screening, while only 32 percent of the Black smoker lung cancer patients were. (It's amazing to me that you can have lung cancer and *still* not be considered eligible for early detection.) Working with a biostatistician, Drs. Aldrich, Grogan, Sandler, and their colleagues ultimately determined that Black Americans had the same lung cancer risk at twenty pack years that other races had after thirty pack years. Their article, called "Evaluation of USPSTF Lung Cancer Screening Guidelines Among African American Adult Smokers," was published in the *Journal of the American Medical Association Oncology.* It recommended that the USPSTF look closely at their screening guidelines and consider whether they were being too conservative in their recommendations for Black Americans.

When the USPSTF met, they reviewed the article and agreed. Not long after, they recommended that *all* twenty-pack-year smokers—not just Black Americans—be screened starting at age fifty. This just shows how MASLAB and other labs like it are doing profound, important work for a population that's not only at risk but has historically been misunderstood and underserved. If Dr. Grogan and his team hadn't had the interdisciplinary focus as well as the specimens and data that make up the mandate of MASLAB, they might not have moved the needle at the USPSTF.

Both before my surgery and six weeks after, a technician at the MASLAB took samples of my blood, then spun it into its components in a centrifuge. He noted which biomarkers were elevated before my surgery, then, six weeks later, compared my post-op levels to see if those same markers dropped after my surgery. Their data, plus the data from the blood samples of all the other lung cancer patients at Vanderbilt who've consented to testing, will help them publish papers that show the relationship between particular blood-based biomarkers and the presence of cancer. In case they need to use the sample of blood later, they'll freeze it at –80 degrees Celsius and put it in the MASLAB, where it can be stored indefinitely.

Years from now, if my blood is needed for additional research, it can be pulled from the bank and tested again.

The ultimate goal is to develop a blood-based test or liquid biopsy for lung cancer as a screening and treatment tool. In an ideal world, blood tests not only determine whether someone has lung cancer, but also how they respond after treatment. If someone has a recurrence, a blood test could provide important information about how to treat the cancer the second time around. Substantial progress is being made, but Dr. Grogan estimates we're a good ten to twenty years before these kinds of tests will be fully approved and in routine use, but he's reassured that this could happen within his lifetime. In his words, "When I die, if I've been a part of helping to expand lung cancer screening and more people have been captured, and I'm a part of contributing in some way . . . for there to be blood tests or liquid biopsies for lung cancer that are used regularly, I will consider that a successful career."

Commercial Multi-Cancer Detection Tests

MASLAB is not the only place that's working hard to develop blood-based biomarker testing for lung cancer. In fact, one of the most exciting, fast-paced areas of cancer innovation lies with a few companies that are combining existing data with machine learning to create blood testing tools that will help diagnose a number of different kinds of cancer. Yes, I know it can be controversial and scary at times, but AI is already revolutionizing diagnostic tools across medicine, giving doctors and researchers more ways to innovate. In fact, tech and medicine go hand in hand to give patients better ways to get the diagnoses and treatments they so desperately need.

Multi-cancer detection (MCD) tests are exactly what they sound like: They are somatic tests done on body fluids or waste products (like blood, urine, stool, or saliva) that can detect any number of cancers. The only cancers that currently have screenings available are cervical, breast, lung, pancreatic, colorectal, and prostate cancer, and MCD hold the promise of helping to diagnose these and other cancers when screening isn't available—or when it's unnecessarily complicated or inaccessible, like lung cancer screenings can be for people who don't meet screening requirements. MCDs are not yet FDA-approved, but some can be ordered by doctors under a set of regulations called the Clinical Laboratory Improvement Act (CLIA). Those that are approved under this act are the GRAIL Galleri tests and the Cancerguard and Cologuard tests, both of which are actively working toward securing FDA approval in the near future. Nodify is another blood test working toward approval as well.

MCDs work on the assumption that all cancers share a molecular basis. While Cancerguard looks at both cancer-specific protein biomarkers and DNA from cancer-driving genes, Galleri only aims to find circulating DNA that's been shed by cancer cells. Both look for approximately fifty different kinds of cancer—many of which don't have recommended screenings—and while they're not available without a doctor's prescription, they have available telemedicine doctors who can prescribe them for you. Costing around $700–900, the test shows up in the mail, and then you go to a lab for a blood draw. Once you've given your sample, you mail it off, and your results come back within two weeks.

Just remember that no MCD will predict your future genetic risk for cancer. While both look at your DNA, they do not reveal particular genetic mutations that may make it more likely for you to develop cancer. An MCD is a screening tool, not a genetic test. (Mine was negative.)

So, what's stopping MCDs from hitting the mainstream, other than the lack of FDA approval? First, we are still waiting for a mountain of data to figure out their efficacy. There isn't enough available research to see if these tests have reduced cancer mortality rates both for specific cancers and for cancer across the board. Secondly, early data indicates that MCDs produce a large number of false positives—as much as 50 percent in one study.[6] This can lead to unnecessary additional testing and biopsies. Finally, because the studies around MCDs were completed using subjects of all ages, both with cancer and without, it poses a challenge for the USPSTF to recommend age guidelines. In short, the data is still new. However, this is such a rapidly evolving field, with tremendous amounts of money and need driving them, so it may be one of those situations where you blink and suddenly the landscape of blood-based biomarker testing has changed. At the very least, we hope this is the case for some cancers. But I know it may be a long time coming for lung cancer, which can be a difficult cancer to screen, for reasons Dr. Grogan was gracious enough to explain.

Why Blood-Based Biomarker Testing for Lung Cancer is Complicated

What's holding us back from having blood tests that can easily detect the possible presence of lung cancer? Why doesn't lung cancer have its own Cologuard (a test that determines the presence of hemoglobin or altered DNA in stool, pointing to the possibility of colon cancer) or its own PSA test, like you'd take for prostate cancer? According to Dr. Grogan, it's because lung cancer cells are just *different.*

> The hard part about lung cancer is that [unlike other cancers] it's not made up of one cell type. If you look at the markers that can be seen in blood tests for other cancers, there's CEA (carcinoembyonic

> antigen, a protein found on the surface of some cancer cells) for colon and some others cancers, PSA (prostate-specific antigen) for prostate, and CA-125 (protein cancer antigen 125) for ovarian. Most of those cancers are predominantly one cell type, and they come from the same line of cells. Lung cancer has more than five major cell types.

I knew where my adenocarcinoma originated: in the epithelial cells that line the surface of my lungs. But, like Dr. Grogan said, there are many other cells associated with lung cancer as well, including neuroendocrine and squamous cells. "So, finding one biomarker that works is hard," Dr. Grogan continued. "We're working on trying to find multiple different types of biomarkers that will work."

Thinking back on the genetic testing I had after my mom's cancer, I wondered whether there was any future in genetic testing or whether scientists' efforts were best spent looking at other kinds of biomarkers. Dr. Grogan's answer was a short one. "Right now, they're not good enough because there's so many different types of lung cancer. And there's not enough good blood and tissue banks to help provide the specimens for that. We're trying to fix that problem. It's a tough problem. That's one of the reasons why I went into it, because I like solving tough problems."

Remembering Susan

Dr. Grogan is right; lung cancer is a tough problem to solve. But people are tougher, especially those who've battled lung cancer. We are strong and determined and won't stop till we find a cure. One of the people I most wish I had with me on this journey is the late Susan Wojcicki, who was the older sister of my dear friend Anne Wojcicki. Susan passed away from lung cancer in the summer of 2024 at the age of fifty-six, and I want to honor her memory and the cause she championed until her death.

Susan Wojcicki was the oldest of three sisters who grew up on the campus of Stanford University with a dad who was a professor and a mom who was a journalist. Susan and her sisters were only a few years apart in age, and, as Anne said, "she was the adult in the room. Susan was very responsible . . . she was very much the big sister and also the peacekeeper. Susan was the leader of the tribe." She was also smart—really, really smart. She graduated from Harvard University and earned two graduate degrees before becoming employee #16 at Google. Not long into her time at Google, she recommended that the company snatch up a start-up online video service called YouTube. She helped oversee the purchase and became CEO of YouTube in 2014. Also, along the way she had five children. Susan was good at pretty much everything.

(Continued . . .)

In late 2022, Susan was supposed to go on a walk with a friend but canceled because she was having hip pain. She ran a few miles a day, so she assumed she'd pulled a muscle and didn't think much of it. When the pain continued longer than it should have, Susan decided to get an MRI. It revealed that she had non-small cell lung cancer, and it had metastasized into her bones.

At this late stage, Susan's cancer was inoperable and likely irreversible. It was also a huge mystery to everyone. Susan always ate healthy foods, did not smoke, and had no family history of lung cancer. When she tested her house for radon, the report came back clean, and when she did genetic testing, she had no heritable genetic mutation that might have caused it. When the oncologist listened to her lungs, they sounded perfect (isn't that familiar?). Here was a healthy, highly successful woman (and mom) who'd done everything to keep herself healthy, and with no symptoms other than hip pain, she was suddenly in a fight for her life. It was inconceivable to everyone around her, but it was the hard reality she had to face.

Susan stepped down from her position at YouTube and, as Anne said, "became the CEO of her own cancer." Her cancer was too far advanced for surgery, so she investigated clinical trials and many of the amazing cellular therapies that are available today. In the end, nothing worked, and Susan passed away from lung cancer on August 9, 2024. She is deeply missed by everyone who knew and loved her.

In a few chapters, I'll talk more about the work Susan did before she passed away and that her sister, Anne, now continues to help stop this disease, but, for now, I want to honor her memory. Susan didn't beat cancer, but it never dimmed her incredible spirit or the energy she brought to her family, friends, and colleagues. On behalf of lung cancer survivors everywhere, we are so grateful to Susan.

Chapter Twelve

The Future of Screening

Artificial intelligence (AI) is powering innovation across the creative, industrial, logistical, medical, and technology sectors, and it's developing more and more each day. It is fascinating to follow how it is helping in the healthcare industry. Drs. Kim Sandler and Eric Grogan walked me through the many ways AI has become a powerful complement to the diagnosis and treatment of lung cancer, from the radiologists' readings to the surgery to the future detection of disease.

Pathology

One of the first ways that machine learning is revolutionizing lung cancer treatment involves diagnostics. AI has become another set of eyeballs, but it's one that is backed by data and powered by algorithms.

When radiologists find a nodule on a scan, they have a very specific set of recommendations about how to study it based on its morphology (shape and structure) and its size. If there's a nodule, they may ask another radiologist for a second opinion. If there's clearly no nodule present on a scan, they move on. AI can act as a third opinion, giving a clearer diagnostic picture that humans simply don't have the eyes to see.

AI also works on the basis of algorithms that track patterns based on scientific studies, and, like a trusted research assistant, it points those out to the radiologist. A scan with no suspicious nodules may be flagged by AI because the machine has looked at tens of thousands of studies and understands that a particular combination of health history, biomarkers, age, smoking history, or any other risk factor may point to their likelihood of developing lung cancer. The machine can synthesize the data to uncover the pattern, and the pattern can then be used to put the most high-risk scans at the top of the pile.

With AI, radiology isn't just about the eyeballs. It's also about the data.

Kim explains one example of how this works in her day-to-day:

> So, when I'm reading a CT scan, there's a machine learning program running in the background that tells me whether or not it thinks there's a blood clot.

> And what's nice is that if it does think there's one, it'll flag it so that that study doesn't sit on my list until later in the day. It's like, no, no, look at this one now.

All that being said, it is crucial to understand the importance of not only relying on AI but also using physicians to empower it. For example, a machine may tailor its algorithm based on the data coming out of a particular scanner. If you've scanned more people with one device, the machine learning algorithm may be weighing data from a scanner more than studying what it's actually seeing. A radiologist has to factor in all of these considerations when they look at scans, balancing the learned knowledge of the machine with the expertise of a trained physician.

Hopefully in the near future, radiologists from institutions across the country and around the world will be able to combine their data on large population groups to streamline the work that AI is already doing. The more information there is to work from, the deeper the levels of care. The simple truth is we can't keep missing these hard-to-find cancers, and AI is there as a powerful tool to supplement.

Radiomics

Radiomics is an AI tool that extracts large amounts of data from radiological images (CT, MRI, and PET scans) and breaks them down into their pixels and voxels (which are essentially pixels in 3D). This allows radiologists to look at scans more closely than with the naked eye. It uncovers hidden patterns to help prevent disease progression and improve responses and outcomes. As Dr. Grogan put it, "If I look at a CT scan, I can see the spot and I can see kind of how it looks. But the radiomic tools go in and they super-analyze it, pulling out features that the human eye couldn't detect." These features are saved and stored in large databases that doctors and scientists can then use to help diagnose and treat cancer, as well as make predictions for the cancer's likelihood of growth and spread, its possible hereditary characteristics, and more. Just like all improvements in imaging, it's a tremendously helpful tool that will likely only improve as time passes.

The current challenge, highlighted in a July 2025 journal article in *Clinical Radiology*, is getting the technology into the doctors' hands. As the study says, "Implementation remains limited due to challenges in data standardization, validation, and health-care integration, requiring cross-center result replication. Despite their potential, radiomics methods are not yet fully integrated into precision medicine, though some, like the RPV score in ovarian cancer, are in final prospective studies for incorporation."[1] Thankfully, AI is constantly evolving and we are getting closer and closer to being able to use it more and more.

23andMe (and Anne)

I met Anne Wojcicki when I was in my twenties, working in San Francisco. Though we lost touch as we went different ways with marriage and children and cross-country moves, we found each other again living in Montana during the COVID-19 pandemic. I had to remind her of our past partying days, and that brought us right back to being fast friends. We kicked off where we left off with too much fun.

Anne's sister, Susan, who I talked about in the last chapter, passed away from lung cancer in August 2024. Just thirteen months later, I was diagnosed with it. Anne was one of the first people I called, and she has been a wise, steady presence through every twist and turn of my lung cancer journey.

Anne started her career as a health-care investor and analyst, focusing on biotech companies. In 2006, she decided to pivot, and she took her skills as an investor and her knowledge of health care and cofounded a genetic testing company called 23andMe. The premise was simple: You mail in a sample of your saliva to the company, and they map your genome and send you the results of your ancestry and genetic predispositions for certain diseases.

When Anne learned her sister had lung cancer in 2022, she says she immediately took a week off and called sixty people with expertise in cancer research and treatment. That's exactly what I did (mostly) but Anne took it a step further by starting a thorough genetics study. As she watched her sister battle lung cancer, she searched for ways that she and Susan could help innovate research and treat the disease. The Wojcicki sisters decided to start a nonprofit research institute that would directly benefit lung cancer patients and their families. Anne resigned as CEO in 2025 as 23andMe struggled in bankruptcy. But later that year, her nonprofit purchased 23andMe, helping put Anne back in the driver's seat, where she was able to launch a program called the Lung Cancer Genetics Study. Her sister's memory was and is an integral part of this initiative.

The Lung Cancer Genetics Study's goal is to build a genetic database of lung cancer patients so that they can track heritable risk factors. Study participants submit a saliva sample much like they would with 23andMe, and they receive a genetic analysis in return. Over the course of their treatment, they can respond to surveys about the progress of their disease, and that information will help supplement the genetic results. The goal is to understand how tumor mutations, including heritable mutations, and lifestyle and environmental factors interact to better understand what kind of risk factors are at play. Anne's goal is to have ten thousand participants to study to help improve lung cancer detection and treatments.

AI and Precision Medicine

There are mountains of research and data concerning all types of cancer—spanning decades and crossing borders—and sorting through all of it is next to impossible. A biotech company called Tempus, however, is trying to solve this problem. Tempus has amassed what they say is the world's largest library of clinical and molecular data on cancer, and it uses AI to mine it for answers, then combines it with genome sequencing to help formulate plans to treat patients. Tempus's aim is to offer each patient an individualized road map for treatment based on their particular genetic makeup rather than a one-size-fits-all approach that doesn't take into account the differences in their DNA. This extremely tailored approach is called "precision medicine." Think of it this way: While a company like Anne's is trying to track the genetic reasons why someone might get lung cancer, Tempus and other companies like it (including Signatara and Gardent 360) are seeing how genetics can influence treatment.

These companies take the available data about certain diseases, including genomic data, and aggregate it in such a way that a doctor can weigh the clinical information they have about a patient against the historical data gleaned through machine learning. With a body of knowledge and a patient's particular situation, a physician can make real-time decisions about a course of treatment rather than simply using the knowledge they have in their head.

AI can be a set of eyeballs *and* another brain, and companies like Tempus offer precision oncology based on each patient and informed by mountains of genomic data.

Erik Hale, Two-time Lung Cancer Survivor, Stage 3A, Colorado

When I was thirty years old, I noticed during my workouts that it was getting a lot harder for me to breathe. I had childhood asthma that had gone away a little bit, but I still had inhalers. I was hitting my inhaler a lot—like every 15 to 30 minutes—and it wasn't really doing anything. It got to the point where I was just walking on a treadmill and could barely keep myself up and get enough breath. I thought, *This is just not right. Something is up.* So, I went to my general care practitioner at the time, out in California, and they ended up doing a chest X-ray. The doctor said, "Oh yeah, it looks like you have walking pneumonia, so we're going to prescribe you all these meds, and it'll take care of it."

She sent me home.

A few weeks to maybe a month passed. I did the round of antibiotics, and it was not getting better. I was a preschool teacher at the time, and I'm in the classroom with active kids and barely keeping it together. So, I go back

(Continued . . .)

and I say, "It's not getting better. We've got to do something else." They do some other tests and say, "Actually, we think it's a fungal infection. What we're going to do is give you this whole lineup of antifungal meds."

They sent me on my way.

Long story short, it was three to four months of misdiagnosis until I finally went back and was like, "I'm not okay, guys." What I didn't know at the time was to push harder and advocate for myself, which is one big lesson I took from this whole experience. I just thought that doctors know what's best. They're going to take care of me. Now I tell other people that if they don't feel right, push the doctor for more help. If they're not giving you that help, fire them and get another one who will.

They finally did a needle biopsy in my back because there was something cloudy on an X-ray. And when they did the needle biopsy, it came back positive for lung cancer, and they determined it was stage 3A already. I was obviously shocked, at thirty as a nonsmoker. My mom had breast cancer and my grandfather had skin cancer at some point late in life. But no one had had lung cancer. I thought, *What are you talking about? Are you serious?* I was also upset because I had been asking for help with this for a long time already. It could have been the difference in staging for me. During my treatment in 2013, the five-year survival rate for stage 3A lung cancer was 4 percent.

As soon as they diagnosed me with lung cancer, I was told to come back the following week and start on radiation treatments for five weeks. Then I'd go through chemo for six weeks. Then they'd remove half my left lung in surgery.

At the time, my now-wife and I were just living together. We were boyfriend and girlfriend. When I found out, I was at the preschool on my lunch break. My wife was at work down in Mountain View two hours away. I didn't want to call her and tell her this, obviously. When she got home that evening, I sat her down and said, "Hey, look, this is what they're telling me." And when I gave her the diagnosis, legit, the first response she had was: "We're getting married."

I think it takes a unique individual to respond that way. We'd only been dating maybe a year and a half or two years at the time. A lot of people faced with that kind of thing would have just been like, "I'm out," and I wouldn't blame anybody who said that. After I got diagnosed, I had a lot of friends fall off. I just stopped hearing from them. I don't blame them, because this is too real for some people. But my wife, she was such a strong foundation for me during that time. She's been that all these years, and we're still together.

The treatment plan was a whirlwind at the time, but I thought, *Well, I don't have any other options.* Radiation was four to five weeks and then chemo was six. People have horror stories about how that goes for them. I don't want to say it was a breeze, but compared to what other

(Continued . . .)

people experienced, I had very little symptoms. I lost my hair. I had deep fatigue, but that was about it.

When I had the lobectomy to remove half of my left lung a week or two later, that was the real wake-up call. It was an eight-hour surgery. When I woke up, I thought, *Oh, this is a level of pain that I've never felt before.* The only way I can describe it is like having your soul removed from your body.

Here I'm lying in bed, bald, barely able to breathe, hooked up with tubes draining blood out of my body. I went from this robust guy to not even being able to walk to the bathroom by myself. I was in the hospital nine days after surgery because I was so weak and in so much pain. When I did get sent home, it took me almost a whole year to get back to normal-ish life. Within that year, I started to go back to the gym, but I was barely lifting the lightest possible weight and just getting movement.

The other problem was that I had so much pain from that surgery that they put me on a very, very high dose of oxycodone and morphine throughout that year when I was recovering. We eventually had to drop the morphine because I couldn't keep food down anymore.

Once that year had passed, I was like, "I can't be on these meds anymore. I have to stop this." I was barely myself at that point. I had two weeks of the worst withdrawals of my life and no one really prepared me for that. No one told me that would happen or how to navigate it.

All these things cascaded out of what I had been through. But I'm glad that I had the wherewithal to know that if I didn't get off this stuff, I never would.

In 2019, I had a recurrence, and they didn't do any other treatments other than an arthroscopic surgery to remove a bunch of mediastinal lymph nodes in the middle of my chest. Two of the eight they removed had cancer. I found out I have an EGFR mutation, and if heaven forbid cancer ever comes back, I know there are few drugs out there that I could actually use. But since 2019, no cancer. I get CT scans and blood work done, but only once a year now because I'm so far out.

I have had multiple oncologists tell me my story is unheard of. There's no way I should still be here. There are lot of people I've met along the way that had diagnoses similar or even less serious than mine that have passed away now. I don't know whether it's because of God, fate, or the random chaos of the universe, but I'm unbelievably lucky to still be here.

In the early days, I still thought I didn't have a chance to survive, so I focused mostly on just enjoying my life. My wife and I would have started having kids, but my father died when I was twelve. I knew what it was like to grow up without a parent, and I didn't want that for any future kids that I had. I wanted to be able to be there for them.

(Continued . . .)

Then I had the recurrence in 2019, and after that, I started thinking, *Well, I might live. I think I might have to plan the rest of my life.*

I had my first child when I was thirty-nine, and my second two years later. What lung cancer has shown me is that I have to live with intention and try to do the things that scare me. I got very into fitness and tried to see how far I could push myself with that. I advanced my career at work, and I've been an instructional and graphic designer at a tech company for eleven years. And I'm an indie author. I've got these stories to tell, and I want to tell them.

I also work with the GoTo Foundation. Every year the GoTo Foundation does a summit where they have lung cancer survivors come out to Washington and meet representatives and senators from our states. We tell them about lung cancer to try to reduce the stigma that lung cancer is just a smoker's disease. They love me because I was a young nonsmoker when this happened. We highlight the need for more funding and research, that lung cancer is one of the deadliest cancers because it's just detected so late.

When I was first diagnosed, I didn't have a lot of treatment options. I'm proud to say that I feel like I've had a hand in those numbers getting better over time. It just showed me to take these risks, do these things. The only person who can limit me is myself. And I'm already on my second or third of my nine lives if I'm a cat, right? So, I might as well take the shot. I wouldn't wish the pain and fear of cancer on anyone, but the growth that I've had from it and the opportunities I've had for advocacy has been worth it. And I think that's part of my view on life is just when something negative happens to you, you better do something with it because otherwise what's the point, right?

Chapter Thirteen

Nonsurgical Treatments for Lung Cancer

When I first found out about Susan Wojcicki's cancer, I didn't fully appreciate the enormity of what her family went through. During her illness, they had to navigate a terrible tragedy, help her wrap up her work, care for her five children, and be with her as she endured grueling treatments. Susan did not receive an LDCT for early detection, and she found her cancer after it had already spread. Susan was healthy and in the prime of her life, and the screening guidelines did not include her. Despite Susan being in a position to get the help she needed, there was very little she could do in the face of lung cancer. In the end, the lung cancer won, and her family, friends, colleagues, and the world had to let her go.

It's simply not fair. Susan's family should still have her just like my family has me. My kids saw me in the hospital for a few days and then at home resting. They don't understand how lucky we are, and it is not something I take lightly.

There's been no chemotherapy or radiation for me (yet) or any of the other treatments that many people like Susan undergo. I saw my oncologist a month after my surgery, when I got my results from my biomarker tests. Yep, they have you wait to see the oncologist. It turns out, oncologists are not the one-stop shop for all things cancer related. The oncologist is "the cancer person," and if your cancer is cut out and your margins are clear, there may be little for the oncologist to do. As my surgeon said, he wields the knife while the oncologist wields the poison.

The oncologist walked me through the stage of my cancer and how he views treatments differently for everyone. Below, I outline what we discussed and what I have come to understand could have been my reality if a scan hadn't found my lung cancer so early.

Staging

As with any cancer, lung cancer is classified into stages based on how much it has progressed and where the cancer cells are located. While every person and every cancer is different, physicians typically determine a cancer's stage after looking at a biopsy of a mass and determining whether cancer cells are in your lymph nodes. Staging helps direct what a treatment plan will entail and gives hints about your prognosis. Knowing a cancer's stage won't tell you how many years you can survive with the disease, but it will help provide a road map for you and your doctors.

The system used for determining a stage is often called the TNM classification system, and it entails:

- T: Tumor size and location
- N: N is for nodes, as in the lymph nodes. Determining if cancer cells have spread to the lymph nodes in the chest cavity will help classify your cancer.
- M: M is for metastasis, meaning the other organs to which the cancer has spread.

Using this information, a team of physicians can then determine whether a cancer falls into one of several stages. The stages I describe below are specifically for non-small cell lung cancer, which makes up about 80 to 85 percent of cases. As you might remember, it's what I had, and while it's less aggressive than small cell lung cancer, it often strikes nonsmokers and grows without causing obvious symptoms. Never-smokers aren't eligible for screening, so it's also the toughest kind of cancer to catch early. NSCLC is staged as limited, meaning it is confined to one lung and/or the lymph nodes in the chest cavity, or it can be extensive, meaning it's spread to both lungs and/or the other organs.

1. **Stage 0:** In stage 0 NSCLC, the cancer is confined to the top lining of the lungs or bronchus.
2. **Stage I:** Stage I means that the cancer has not spread to the lymph nodes.
3. **Stage II:** This stage indicates that the cancer is larger than stage I and has spread to the lymph nodes but not the other organs.
4. **Stage III:** The cancer is larger than stage II and has spread to the lymph nodes but not other organs.
5. **Stage IV:** In stage IV, the cancer has spread to other organs.

The cancer is further classified according to its size. For instance:

- **Stage 1A1:** The tumor is one centimeter or smaller
- **Stage 1A2:** The tumor is between one and two centimeters.
- **Stage 1A3:** The tumor is between two and three centimeters.
- **Stage 1B:** The tumor is between three and four centimeters. Or the tumor is four centimeters or less and:

- Growing in the bronchus but hasn't reached the point where the windpipe splits into the two bronchi.
- Cancer cells are found on the pleura, which is the tissue that surrounds the lungs.
- The tumor is blocking the airways.

I learned at my oncology appointment that my cancer wasn't over four centimeters, like we'd thought at my CT, but rather two centimeters. That made it stage IA2.

Over two-thirds of people with my type of lung cancer present (meaning they get a diagnosis) with stage III and stage IV. As Dr. Grogan said, "Most of them go right to the oncologist. I never get the opportunity to even evaluate them surgically. Our treatments and therapies for people in these later stages aren't as good as some of the other diseases, but even in most cancers, stage III and stage IV is a challenge."

Susan Wojcicki was stage IV, while I had a tumor that was small and hadn't spread. At Dr. Grogan's "tumor board meeting," he and his team carefully analyzed my results and determined I could have surgery. When I visited my oncologist, it was time for me to learn if we'd follow up my surgery with chemotherapy, radiation, or another kind of treatment. Would I lose my hair? Would my kids finally see that I really, truly was sick with something that could change the course of our lives? No matter what, I knew I was lucky, but I soon learned just how lucky I was. As I sat waiting for my oncologist to propose a treatment plan for me, I knew the options I might have to consider were as follows:

- **Chemotherapy:** Chemotherapy is like a nuclear bomb, killing everything in its path, including cancer cells and often healthy cells as well. A patient might have chemotherapy to shrink a tumor's size before surgery (termed neoadjuvant treatment) or to kill any remaining cancer cells after surgery (termed adjuvant therapy). Chemotherapy may be given in combination with radiation and is often given to late-stage patients to keep the cancer growth at bay. It may be given in chunks of time lasting three to four weeks and sometimes longer, and it does not require a hospital stay.
- **Radiation:** Radiation involves powerful cancer-killing X-rays that are targeted directly at a tumor. Less often, radioactive material may be placed directly inside a tumor so that it kills the tumor from the inside out. Like chemotherapy, radiation can be given before surgery to shrink a tumor or when surgery isn't an option.
- **Immunotherapy:** There are several kinds of immunotherapy, but all of them harness the

power of your body's immune system to kill the cancer cells. The immune system uses what are called T cells to kill viruses and cancer cells, but the unstable cancer cells often adapt by developing proteins that silence the immune response. Given through an IV, injection, or shot, immunotherapy drugs will block checkpoint proteins (like PD-1/PD-L1) that cancer uses to hide, effectively allowing the immune system to do its job. There is also a more aggressive type of immunotherapy called adoptive T-cell therapy (ACT) which is currently available in clinical trials, as well as CAR T-cell therapy, which genetically engineers a patient's T cells to fight their cancer cells. Lastly, there are FDA-approved therapeutic cancer vaccines for prostate and bladder cancer, which are technically not vaccines but rather immunotherapies that target cancer proteins or boost the immune response against those proteins. It's important to note that the FDA has not yet approved this form of treatment for lung cancer, though it is available in other countries. I met one woman who visits Germany every four weeks, gets a vaccine-type shot, and travels back home. She plans to do this for over a year, when her course of vaccine immunotherapy is complete.

- **Targeted Drug Therapy:** This class of treatment works by stopping cell growth. This can be done by targeting biomarkers that help a tumor grow, blocking the blood vessel cells that feed a tumor, or by altering a tumor's tissue or environment. Like chemotherapy, targeted drug therapy is a systemic (rather than local) treatment, but unlike chemotherapy, the risk to healthy cells is low.

When I sat down with my oncologist, he pointed out the results from my biomarker testing indicating that I have a rare mutation called EGFR Exon 20 insertion. EGFR tells cancer cells to grow, and EGFR inhibitors are a targeted drug therapy that blocks that signal. My oncologist brought up one issue: EGFR inhibitors haven't been particularly effective with my particular mutation.[1] In addition, some of the immunotherapy drugs my oncologist might have considered in other, more advanced cases hadn't even been tested on stage I and II lung cancers. They've only been given to patients in the later stages of the disease. While they've shown promising results, they also come with major side effects including pneumonitis, an inflammation of the lungs that presents like pneumonia.

Guess what's really not good if you're missing part of a lung? An inflammation of the lung that presents like pneumonia!

So, what are my marching orders from here on out? My oncologist has put me on what he calls "aggressive surveillance." I will have my lungs CT scanned every three months and regularly undergo bloodwork that will examine my biomarkers indicating any major changes. If there are changes, we can consider altering the course of treatment or continue monitoring me.

"You caught it in stage I," my oncologist said. "The five-year survival rate for people in stage I is ninety percent, so we can monitor your lungs rather than filling you with drugs that might cause unnecessary side effects and haven't necessarily been proven to work."

"What happens if it comes back?" I asked, afraid that what he might say next was definitely going to be worse than "aggressive surveillance."

"Your lung capacity is very strong right now," he said. "In fact, you could live without your right lung. So, we might consider another surgery if it comes back. As you know, surgery is the most effective treatment in the early stages. After that, it is much trickier and harder on the body."

I breathed a sigh of relief.

"After a few years of what we hope will be clear scans, you can go in for a scan every six months. And then ultimately, you'll only get them once a year for the rest of your life."

I closed my eyes and thought of Susan Wojcicki. Then I remembered all the people, like Susan, who caught their cancers in the late stages, when it was too late for surgery, so they had to move on to other therapies. Tens of thousands of those people hadn't been eligible for insurance-paid LDCT scans, which are the most effective way to detect cancer, so tumors had grown quietly in their lungs, often without any symptoms. When they were finally diagnosed, they were fighting an uphill battle. Their children saw them without hair or throwing up, and many of those same kids had to say goodbye to their parents when they passed. Every doctor I'd spoken to, from Eric to Kim to my own father, had told me that if I'd waited six months, my tumor may have been inoperable. In fact, chances are it would have been fatal. I'd dodged that bullet using readily available technology. It had all been *so* simple (despite my anxiety surrounding getting that MRI scan). So, what's holding us back from offering lung screening to each and every American who wants it?

I'd soon discover the answer is anything but straightforward or easy.

Chapter Fourteen

Why Don't We Screen More People?

Hopefully, by now you see the big problem we have on our hands: Lung cancer is on the rise in populations where it never was before, particularly never-smoker women. This has happened despite huge efforts to reverse smoking rates in this country, and now doctors, scientists, advocates, and experts are stumped. We've put warning labels on cigarettes, ended tobacco advertising, banned smoking in public areas, started a national lung cancer screening program, and made efforts to limit radon and air pollution in our cities and our homes. Smoking rates have plummeted, and lung cancer rates with it, but each and every year, more never-smoking women like me come down with lung cancer.

This is a young woman's health crisis.

Clearly, the easiest way to reverse this trend is to screen more people. We can improve treatments, identify biomarkers, and pioneer blood tests that can pinpoint your risk, but if we don't want people to succumb to cancer, we must catch it early. Lung cancer does not have to be and should not be a death sentence.

Downsides of Screening

Low-dose CT scans do carry risks, though they're minimal. But everyone should weigh what they feel comfortable with versus the many benefits that they can convey.

The first risk is radiation. CTs, X-rays, and nuclear medicine (like the PET-CT scan Kim's dad gave me, when he discovered my cancer cells were "on fire") use ionizing radiation, which penetrates tissue to give you a clear view of your organs. This radiation can damage DNA, and while your cells usually repair themselves, there's still a small risk. (Note that MRIs do not use ionizing radiation.)

Every year, about eighty million Americans get some form of medical scan. Additionally, we are all exposed to "background" radiation, including radon in your home or rays from the sun. It's estimated that the average person is exposed to 3 millisieverts (mSv) of this background radiation per year (and the farther away you are from the equator or if you live at a higher altitude, you receive even more of this radiation.) That being said, a low-dose

CT scan exposes a person to only 1.4 millisieverts (mSv) of radiation.

Studies have compared the chances of high-risk individuals getting lung cancer versus the risk of developing cancer from LDCT, and they've determined the benefits of screening outweigh the danger of radiation. A 2017 report states "radiation exposure and cancer risk associated with lung cancer LDCT screening are not negligible, but are acceptable due to the substantial mortality reduction obtained with screening".[1]

I'll give you an example of how radiation exposure affects your cancer risk. In April 2017, a man named Tom Stuker became the world's most frequent flyer by traveling 1.8 million flight miles in fourteen years. That's about 3.7 years of air time. All that traveling at a high altitude—which exposed Stuker to more radiation than he would have faced on the ground—only increased his lifetime risk of contracting a potentially fatal cancer by about 0.5 percent.

Yes, that's right. You can fly for almost four years, absorbing radiation with every passing mile, and still barely move the needle when it comes to your cancer risk. A low-dose CT exposes you to *a lot* less radiation than 1.8 million flight miles do.

One other issue to bear in mind is that once you are over forty, radiation-induced malignancies are less common because people become less radiosensitive as they age. Few people under forty get scanned simply because the likelihood of developing lung cancer before that age is so low. When we scan for lung cancer, we are giving radiation to people whose bodies are equipped to handle the exposure. Truly, there is very little to fear.

One of the other potential risks of screening involve the incidental findings that show up on scans. In addition to histoplasmosis fungus (especially in my part of the country) coccidioidomycosis (common in the southwest) leads to something called "valley fever." When fungal spores are inhaled an infection develops, and the body starts to wall it off to protect itself. That protected bundle is called a granuloma, and during a scan, there

Who Gets Screened—and How Many Lives are Saved

Lung cancer is one of seven cancers you can screen for, yet, among the five major screening programs it's far and away the least utilized. The chart below breaks down the numbers. How many people should get screened for cancer, how many do, how many lives are saved, and how many *should* be saved. As you can see, if we screened for lung cancer at the rate we screen for breast and colorectal cancer, we'd save tens of thousands more lives. (Note: While liver and pancreatic cancer screening is available, it's only for very high-risk individuals and is often only available at specialized locations.)

Cancer Type	Actual Screened (millions)	Should Be Screened (millions)	Gap (Difference, millions)	Screening Rates	Key Notes	Potential Annual Lives Saved	Annual Deaths	Annual Treatment Spending
Lung	2.9–3.5	16.3–19.4	13.4–15.9	~18%	Annual LDCT for ages 50–80, ≥20 pack-year smokers/quits <15 years. Low uptake due to awareness/access barriers	~12,000–26,000 (at 70% uptake; 20% mortality reduction)	~125,000	~$13.5 billion
Breast	32.0 (biennial)	40.0 (biennial)	8.0	~80%	Biennial mammography, ages 40–74. Stable post-COVID; disparities in rural/low-income groups.	~4,000 (at 90% uptake; 20–40% mortality reduction)	~43,000	~$29.8 billion
Colorectal	23.4	34.7	11.3	~67%	Ages 45–75, various tests (e.g. colonoscopy every 10 years). Uptake rose post 2021 guideline update	~26,000 (at 80% uptake; ~30% mortality reduction via polyp removal)	~53,000	~$24.3 billion

Cancer Type	Actual Screened (millions)	Should Be Screened (millions)	Gap (Difference, millions)	Screening Rates	Key Notes	Potential Annual Lives Saved	Annual Deaths	Annual Treatment Spending
Prostate	8.8	23.1	14.3	~38%	PSA testing, ages 55–69, shared decision-making. Rebounded post-2012 decline; higher in Black men	~7,000 (optimized via shared decisions; ~20% mortality reduction)	~35,000	~$12.0 billion
Liver	0.25–0.50 (semiannual)	2.5 (semiannual)	2.0–2.25	~10–20%	Ultrasound/ AFP for high-risk (cirrhosis, hepatitis B or C). Low due to provider gaps; HER alerts help.	~3,000–5,000 (at 75% high-risk uptake; ~30% more early detections, improving survival 20–40%)	~30,000	~$2.5 billion
Pancreatic	0.002–0.005	0.2	0.195–0.198	~1–2.5%	MRI/EUS for high-risk (~200,000 with genetic syndromes). Limited to specialized programs; detects ~%70 early stage	~500–1,000 (at 50% high-risk uptake; ~40% survival improvement in detected cases)	~52,000	~$2.6 billion

are many times when you can't determine whether something is a cancer or an infection. Doctors clearly can't brush finding a nodule under the rug, so—while they may tell you to wait for symptoms to develop, as I was told—there's a strong chance the incidental findings may result in more imaging in three to six months.

Researchers from Northwestern University recently looked at what would happen if we expanded screening to all people aged forty to eighty-five, similar to how we screen for breast and colorectal cancer.[2] They projected that if 70 percent of these people were screened, there would be an estimated sixteen million false positive results every year, and that would cause an additional 1.2 million invasive procedures. Of those procedures 4,900 might cause complications. I know that sounds like a huge number, so let's put it in perspective. Right now, breast cancer screening leads to an estimated 3.3 million false positives and 33,000 biopsies with 500 complications. Universal age-based colorectal screening results in 2.1 million false positives, 420,000 polypectomies, and 3,200 complications. You might argue that breast biopsies are far easier than bronchoscopies, and you're right. But what about polypectomies? Yes, a significant portion are pre-cancerous, but they require a day's worth of prep, which is disruptive and unpleasant, anesthesia, and an invasive procedure. Yet no one is arguing that we limit the number of colorectal screenings we do every year.

Dr. Grogan believes there's a huge opportunity in incidental findings on MRI and CT scans. He told me that radiologists find aortic aneurysms and lymphoma, as well as treatable lung conditions like pneumonia. They also find other cancers, and he estimates that for every ten cancers he finds with LDCTs, one of them isn't lung cancer. Because of that, he believes that incidental findings actually give us an opportunity to improve someone's overall health.

What If We Change How We Do Scans?

The science of radiology is just over one hundred years old, and between X-rays and MRIs and CTs, it's been a productive century that's saved millions of lives. Today, new technology is constantly being developed. As we talked about in chapter 12, AI is speeding these innovations along in huge ways, and every scientist and doctor I've spoken to is thrilled at how much it's already helped them with patient care. Doctors are discovering tumors more easily than they had before, and patient histories and biomarker data are being fed into AI systems that will help them find better care. There's a lot to question about how AI is going to play into our daily lives, but so far, so good with radiology.

Two of the most important concepts in radiology are "signal" and "noise." The "signal" means whatever image you want your eyes to inspect (like my tumor), while the "noise" is every other blurry or distracting image that takes away from what's important. Every scan is judged according to its signal to noise ratio (SNR), and the goal of radiology has always been to get more signal and less noise. One way to do that is to increase the amount of radiation produced by a machine. The more radiation that passes through the body, the more that gets to the detector, and the better your images are.

High-signal images show us more in the picture than we sometimes need to see. The Center for Medicare and Medicaid Services (CMS) sets the bar for all insurance approvals at the federal government level, and they are worried about all the findings that high-signal images might uncover. Any suspicious image might actually be noise, but you won't know unless you biopsy the mass, or if you're lucky, conduct a blood test or liquid biopsy to determine if there are any biomarkers floating in the blood.

Radiologists who study the lungs have a way around this problem, and it's a solution that may help cut down on unnecessary findings. Kim told me that, in lung imaging studies, you can do the opposite of what your gut might tell you, and instead of looking for a better signal, you turn up the noise. "So, I thought what if we make the images worse and that the only thing we see is the lung? Because if you think about the contrast, the air in the lung and the tumor, there's a lot of contrast there. So, we don't actually need great images to find something in the lung."

Lung imaging is similar to other kinds of imaging in this way. Mammograms, for example, use much lower penetrating radiation than CTs because a breast tumor has a similar density to the adjacent breast tissue, and lower penetrability radiation allows radiologists to make this distinction. As Kim says, "The idea with this new low-dose technology or using the same CT technology but with a new protocol is that you could decrease the radiation by a factor of ten, potentially making a chest CT deliver less radiation than a mammogram. Then, your images will be so noisy that the only thing you see is the lung. And so, if it's normal, then you're done."

One step backward, two steps forward. Technology is blazing the way to make it easier and faster to diagnose lung cancer, while human intuition is doing the same by using methods from the past.

Chapter Fifteen

Where Do We Go from Here?

I know I've thrown a lot of facts and figures at you, but if there's anything you've learned from reading this book, there are a few things you should *definitely* remember. (Don't worry, there's no pop quiz.)

1. **Low-dose CTs find lung cancer early**. By Kim's estimation, at Vanderbilt alone, 75 percent of the lung cancers found in their early detection screening program are either stage I or stage II.
2. **When you find lung cancer early, it's likely to be curable.** You can perform surgery, and another treatment if necessary, and continue to screen for it for the rest of your life.
3. **If everyone who was eligible got screened, tens of thousands more Americans would live.** Even

> as I was writing this book, new studies came out that emphasized how powerful early screening is. Researchers at the American Cancer Society looked at what would happen if 100 percent of Americans eligible under the USPSTF's guidelines had a low-dose CT, and they projected that 62,000 deaths from lung cancer could be prevented over five years.[1] That's the population of a small city.

Taken together, what does that mean? *Early screening saves lives.* If you find a nodule, it might scare you half to death, but it won't scare you *to* death. That's an important distinction.

So, how can we screen more people? What can individuals, doctors, hospitals, insurers, and others do to bring more people into clinics and take a close look at their lungs? Over the last decade, screening rates for eligible patients have increased from 5 to 18 percent. This is clearly not high enough, so how can we get to 50, 60, or 70 percent, saving tens of thousands more lives? We also need to expand the eligible patient bucket to include many more people. Eighty percent of women eligible for mammograms get them every year, so it can *definitely* be done. (In addition, most people—in particular, never-smokers—don't need to have their lungs screened annually, but rather about once every three to five years.)

Knowing everything we know about lung cancer prevention and early detection, where do we go from here? To answer that question, I'll introduce you to my new friend, Tiffany.

Tiffany Gowen is the Director of Patient and Family Centered Care at the American College of Radiology (ACR), which is a membership organization for radiologists across the United States. The ACR educates, advocates, and advances best practices, and their goal is to help provide the best patient care to anyone in the United States who receives any kind of scan. At ACR, Tiffany runs their lung cancer screening initiatives, and she is a powerful force in the fight to increase and expand early lung cancer detection in the United States.

I met Tiffany through Kim, and right away I found her energy and passion so infectious that she immediately felt like a good friend. Tiffany's not a radiologist, nor has she had a lung disease, but she started at the ACR as a paper-pushing temp, and, other than eight unhappy months she spent at a consulting firm, she's worked there her whole career.

Today, the job is also deeply personal.

> My brother-in-law passed away from lung cancer at the age of twenty. My husband was a junior in high school, and they got a call. He had a mass in his

> chest, and the NP was like, "You should go home, go get that checked." He was diagnosed in April, and he passed away in September. Six months later, almost to the day, my husband's maternal grandmother passed away from the same type of lung cancer. Now, the thing that's crazy is TJ, my brother-in-law, never smoked a cigarette in his life, whereas his grandmother was a very heavy smoker, but they had the same type of lung cancer. So, that's two very close histories that hit my husband and his family. All that being said, they are not even eligible to be screened because they don't smoke.

Tiffany is now on a mission to change the USPSTF's guidelines so more people can be screened, but she knows that the first hurdle is getting those who are eligible signed up. Right now, there are tens of thousands of Americans who are eligible for lung cancer screenings but, for any number of reasons, can't or won't do it. Tiffany has great ideas on how to take away these barriers to access, and she and I spent time discussing them not long after I had my surgery.

Mobile Screening

The first barrier preventing us from capturing everyone who's eligible for screening starts at the doctor's office. "Lung cancer screening is the only preventative screening that requires you to go see a primary care physician first," Tiffany told me. "You have to have a shared decision-making visit, then you get your referral, then you can have your lung screening. There are hoops that have to be jumped through that no other preventative screening has." With primary care physicians as the gatekeepers, it's hard to do a same-day screening. You can't simply walk into a facility, say you want to get screened, and walk out half an hour later, knowing you'll get your results in a matter of days. If you're not having symptoms—and, remember, few people with early lung cancer have symptoms—you may not be in a rush. Tack on your busy personal schedule and your doctor and clinic's availability, and you may wait weeks or months for a screening. Sometimes, these are weeks and months a person doesn't have. If I'd let my tumor go untreated for six months, it probably would have progressed to stage III or stage IV, and surgery would not have been an option.

Tiffany and the ACR have worked hard to set up mobile screening locations in various places across the country, all of which are staffed with a shared decision-making nurse and primary care doctor who can immediately give a referral. The *New York Times* recently profiled a mobile screening called LUCAS run by the West Virginia University Cancer Institute. In a state with the highest rate of smoking in the country, LUCAS hits two counties a day from March to December. At a cost of $5,000 a day, fully paid with insurance and grants, LUCAS has now screened 4,600 people and detected fifty-five cases of lung cancer. These are people who otherwise may have never received a scan.

Affordability

One of the other major hurdles to screening is affordability. In order to bring eligible people in for lung screenings, cost should never be an issue. While the Affordable Care Act mandates that all insurers fully cover preventive lung cancer screenings for those who meet the guidelines, as I mentioned before, it can cost money to drive to an appointment and take time off work. Enter mobile screenings, which come to you. If mobile screening units were an available option for those concerned about money, affordability would be much less of an issue.

For those of you who aren't currently eligible to be screened, I have good news. In most screening locations in the United States, a low-dose lung CT costs anywhere from $100 to $300. Vanderbilt's lung CT scan recently jumped up to $400 from $150, but, as Kim said, "We're trying to bring it back down to help increase access."

Work with Primary Care Physicians

Another significant barrier to early screening lies with the primary care physicians serving as gatekeepers to the entire screening process. Tiffany is currently working toward her PhD in public health, and one of her major research projects entails a wide-ranging survey of PCPs. Her methodology involves giving these doctors educational information about lung screening, then asking them a series of questions after they've read it. Throughout this process, she's come to believe that many PCPs don't fully understand the criteria for lung screening. Both of my parents and brothers are doctors, so I understand the massive demands of the job. Doctors juggle seeing fifteen to twenty patients a day, sometimes many more, and they are expected to keep up with new studies, recommendations, and guidelines that arrive fast and furious on an almost daily basis. There are simply too many conditions and too many people with them for a doctor to understand every detail about what's available for their patients' preventive health.

So, what do we do? We have to continue to arm both patients and doctors with the latest information about lung cancer screening, and we have to do it often. Tiffany and the ACR work tirelessly to educate PCPs to stay on top of the USPSTF's guidelines and recognize when their patients need to follow them. In addition, they're working to streamline systems that will make a doctor's job easier—something I'll get to later in this chapter.

Make Direct Appeals to Women

As the saying goes, "If you want to get something done, give it to a woman." That's never more true than when it comes to lung cancer screening.

Through their research and advocacy work, Tiffany and others at the ACR have discovered that women who understand the necessity of lung screenings are more likely to influence their family members to get screened. Studies back this up. For example, women tend to better understand details related to health care,[2] and women—especially mothers—shoulder an estimated 80 percent of the family's medical decision-making responsibilities.[3] While I hate to give my fellow women out there one more thing to stay on top of, especially since it was my husband who insisted I have my preventive scan, women are ready, willing, and able to sound the alarm about the necessity of lung cancer screenings. If we arm women with education about lung cancer screening and make it affordable and accessible for them, they will spread the word.

Bundle Lung Cancer Screenings with Mammograms

Studies show that once a woman is diagnosed with breast cancer, she is more likely than the general population to receive a primary lung cancer diagnosis later.[4] The reason for the connection is still unclear, but it's an alarming trend that deals yet another blow to a population that's already at an elevated risk.

When life gives women lemons, however, some of them choose to make lemonade. If there's clearly some mysterious connection between lung and breast cancer, why can't we screen for both at the same time?

In 2021, Kim had the same thought, so she authored a paper that hypothesized that the population of women who are screened for breast cancer may also benefit from lung cancer screenings.[5] In her methodology, she looked at a population of 685 women who had mammograms and discovered that 251 of them were also eligible for lung cancer screenings. Of those 251 women, 25 percent chose to get a lung CT. Their CTs revealed three cases of lung cancer, all of which were treated successfully and resulted in no deaths. But among the 75 percent of eligible women who didn't opt for screening, seven got lung cancer, and five of them died. These findings made her conclusion easy: Women screened for breast cancer who do not get their lungs screened are dying from lung cancer. Yet those who *are* screened have a higher likelihood of living. Clearly, she concluded, "We must capitalize on reducing barriers to improve screening for lung cancer among high-risk women."

As a result of that study, the American College of Radiology created a campaign called "Pink and Pearl" that ties together breast cancer and lung cancer awareness and education. October is Breast Cancer Awareness Month, signified by a pink ribbon, while November is

Lung Cancer Awareness Month, signified by a white ribbon. Through outreach to providers and patients, the ACR's goal is to piggyback lung cancer awareness on the massive and continued success of Breast Cancer Awareness Month.

Over the past several years, Kim and a team of researchers have been working tirelessly on a project called CALM, which stands for Coordinating a Lung Screening with Mammography.[6] Similar to Kim's previous study, they pinpoint women who are coming in for mammograms and determine whether they also qualify for lung screening. If they are eligible, Kim and her team message the woman's provider and urge them to discuss the need for a preventive lung scan as well. So far, the results have been incredible, with a statistically significant increase in uptake of lung screening for eligible women.

Keep Insurance and Hospital Systems Accountable

Creating new programs to bring people in for lung scans holds the potential to increase early detection rates, but many insurance companies and health-care providers already have the tools necessary to do that. They're just using them for other cancers.

There are systems in place today for breast cancer, for example, that don't exist for lung cancer. If I don't get my yearly mammogram, my doctor's office texts me. Then the radiology clinic where I usually receive screenings will also call and text me. Other women I know receive similar reminders from their insurance companies. What's the result? Anecdotally, almost every woman over forty I know, whether she's high risk or not, gets a mammogram. To put a number on that, the CDC reports that, as of 2019, nearly 70 percent of eligible women reported they had a mammogram within the last two years. It's no wonder that there are far fewer breast cancer deaths than lung cancer deaths in the United States.

Thankfully, some health providers already have these systems in place, and they're making a huge difference in capturing eligible patients. For example, since January 2022, the University of Rochester Medical Center has run a multidisciplinary program that uses an algorithm in the hospital network's medical record system to calculate patients' pack years. Each day, providers across all forty-two of U of R's medical offices receive lists of the available screenings for each patient who are coming in for an appointment that day, as well as text messages reminding them not to forget about lung screenings. Today, the medical center enjoys a 72 percent participation rate for lung screenings.[7] In 2023 and 2024, the program detected sixty-three cases of lung cancer, and a full 78 percent were in their early stages of the disease.

This is huge progress—and many lives saved.

Can We Change the Screening Guidelines?

I like dreaming big, and so does everyone I've interviewed for this book. We all envision a day when everyone who's eligible for an early detection blood test or scan makes an appointment and gets into that magical circular tube, then comes out with either good news or a treatment plan that will save their life. I wish so much that this could happen, but it's not realistic. We're never going to reach 100 percent adoption rates for early detection. We also know that even if everyone eligible does get a preventive screening test, others who do not qualify may still pass from lung cancer. That's because our current screening guidelines simply don't capture the lion's share of lung cancers that are out there.

In a recent study out of Northwestern University, researchers looked at one thousand patients who had been diagnosed with lung cancer and learned that only 35 percent of them qualified for screening under the current guidelines.[8] This translates to two thirds of those being diagnosed with lung cancer who do not qualify for screening because they do not have a history of smoking. The vast majority of these individuals were women and never-smokers. Let me repeat that: According to a rigorous scientific analysis done at a top American research institution, a full 65 percent of people with lung cancer weren't offered an inexpensive, easy, widely available tool to detect a disease that may kill them. This is a tragedy.

It's no surprise that the study's authors concluded that we have to expand the screening guidelines. In fact, they estimate that if we adopted a model of universal age-based screening for people forty to eighty-five, we could detect 94 percent of all lung cancers. That would potentially save an additional twenty-six thousand lives each year.

Breast cancer provides a fascinating and convincing window into what might happen if we expand early lung cancer detection. In 1976, the USPSTF didn't exist, but the American Cancer Society did, and they studied all the available research and data about breast cancer detection and determined that for the female over-forty population, mammograms were effective ways to find cancer and treat it early. They made recommendations, doctors and insurers took them to heart, and mammograms became standard practice in the United States for women over the age of forty. The results weren't immediate because adoption took time, but over the years, hundreds of thousands of women's lives—including my mom's—were saved. From 1989 to 2023, breast cancer mortality rates declined by 44 percent, due in large part to early detection.[9]

Other than age and smoking history, **family history** and other risk factors should be highly considered in screening guidelines. Other types of cancer screening factor family history into their early detection programs (colorectal and breast screening), but lung cancer does not. However, there is ample data showing that if one of your close family relatives develops lung cancer, you are at heightened risk of getting the disease yourself. I need to remember this to ensure my children eventually get screened.

Similarly, **environmental exposures** are a driver of lung cancer, but current screening guidelines don't account for radon, cookstoves, secondhand smoke, or work environment factors. Studies reveal that coal miners are at greater risk of lung cancer than the general population, and this risk has risen over the years.[10] But if you're a forty-year-old coal miner who's spent five days a week for twenty years breathing in coal dust—yet you've never smoked a cigarette—you're still not eligible for early screening. This makes no sense. Lung cancer screening guidelines should absolutely, positively take into account the fact that certain environmental exposures increase your risk.

Dr. Grogan told me he and his colleague, epidemiologist Dr. Stephen Deppen, are now amassing data about environmental exposures using resources from the US Department of Veterans Affairs health system.

> My colleague Steve and I have a $1.2 million grant. And the goal of that grant is to look at veteran exposures [and how they increase your risk]. And should

> those be included in the lung cancer screening guidelines? So, we've gone to the VA national database and first started to quantify veterans' smoking histories, which, as we previously mentioned, is hard. We've also pulled out everybody with exposures, and we started to look at their lung cancer risk. Where are we going to expand the guidelines? Exposures? Like, for people that have exposures other than smoke, radon, asbestos? Right now, [the only environmental exposure the guidelines account for is] smoking. What about burn pits? We're still amassing that data to tell whether there are burn pit exposures . . . when many veterans were in Afghanistan, they were near burn pits.

People exposed to the chemical dust produced by the 9/11 terrorist attacks should be eligible for lung cancer screening. Our service members—who fought valiantly around the world—frequently stood next to massive, open-air burn pits, which incinerated plastic, chemicals, and other kinds of waste, and they inhaled their toxic fumes. Yet they're not eligible for early screening. Thankfully, Eric and Steve are working to amass data that will reveal these veterans' lung cancer rates. They plan to publish a paper on it, and if all goes well, the USPSTF will take it into account and expand screening.

With the advent of AI, there's a huge opportunity to combine the kind of data Kim, Eric, and other researchers compile with historical records so we can highlight trends. This may impact not only *who* gets screened, but how often they do. Dr. Grogan agreed with me. "We have an opportunity to combine somebody's clinical history with machine learning algorithms that can predict the development of lung cancer," he said. "And we can pull all of that data together to tell someone, okay, you've had this test. You don't have a very high-risk profile and your imaging looks great. You can come back in three years, whereas someone else may come back in one year."

Kim wholeheartedly (and independently from Eric) was on board with this analysis. She even argued that in order to get the data we need to determine who should be screened, we need to offer screening to *everyone*, then see how the prediction of lives saved compares to the costs and risks from incidental findings.

"I'm so tired of parsing all of these different high-risk populations because there's so much crossover," she said. "[For example,] you can be an Asian woman who has a family history. Let's just offer screening to everyone and then let's find out what the [data says]. Because if we screen everyone, we probably don't need to screen everyone every year. So, what should that interval look like, and how can we use all of the data that's available to us?

Family history, ideally a blood-based biomarker, if we can find one that we feel really confident with."

Kim goes on to point out how the information we have from imaging—not just from research studies—helps determine people's risk factors. Basically, when you get screened, you create a historical record for yourself that can be analyzed using machine learning to see what your risk factors are.

"And then also, our imaging allows us to do risk prediction using the images themselves," Kim said. "And what somebody's likelihood is of developing lung cancer in the next five or six years depending on their imaging . . . they can take a CT scan and say, your risk of developing lung cancer over the next six years is X. I prefer the idea of combining somebody's clinical history, their demographics, with the images."

Universal age-based screening—starting around forty—would allow researchers to pull together the necessary data to analyze trends. Obviously, lung cancer mortality rates would go down, but would costs go up? What about incidental findings? We can't know either of these things until we have a clear, full picture of who's getting sick.

Universal age-based screening might have another, unintended result as well. If smokers and never smokers alike are allowed to get screened, the smokers might not feel so stigmatized. Sitting in a waiting room, no one will know who smokes and who doesn't. As Tiffany says, "I actually think that if we opened it up to everyone, we would do a much better job enrolling people who meet current guidelines because it would not be so stigmatizing. They wouldn't feel like they're being judged in some way."

Level the playing field and everyone wins.

Take It to Washington

We need federal, state, and local governments to rally behind early screening as well. Governments allocate and issue public funds, create laws, and develop awareness campaigns that open people's eyes to real problems, and lung cancer is at the top of that list. I was shocked to read a 2017 American Lung Cancer report called the Lung Health Barometer, which revealed that a full 87 percent of Americans have no familiarity with low-dose CTs. Even worse, 84 percent of high-risk patients are in the dark about scans.

This must be fixed.

Dr. Susan Blumenthal said, "We need the government to conduct major education campaigns about lung cancer, emphasizing how it affects women to ensure that women become aware that this disease is the leading cause of cancer death for them. If they're smokers particularly, but if they're nonsmokers, too. A national campaign must be implemented like we did for breast cancer, cholesterol reduction, and depression. Through education and policy changes, the government, working with NGOs and the private sector, brought down smoking rates from 45 percent of all adults in the 1950s to 12 percent of adults today. That's a significant reduction."

If anyone should know, it's Rear Admiral Susan Blumenthal. When she worked as US Assistant Surgeon General and the First Deputy Assistant Secretary for Women's Health, thirty years ago, she cochaired the president's breast cancer initiative. One day she called up the director of the CIA, the head of NASA, and a general at the Department of Defense, and she asked them if they would send their top imaging scientists to a conference she was organizing with our nation's top radiologists. The goal was to harness these agencies' knowledge and technology for detecting missiles and visualizing the surface of Mars to radically transform and modernize screening for breast cancer, a disease Susan's mother had died from. This program, called "Missiles to Mammograms" helped launch digital mammography to the masses and was at the forefront of applying AI in radiology. This fueled computer assisted diagnosis, which is now being used in detection of lung and other cancers.

Grassroots Efforts

The government can't solve everything. We have so much power as individuals to make change. Some of us are business owners, and some of us like to wear ribbons, make signs, and demonstrate or march. Others of us just like to talk to our kids and friends about what we've been through, what we've witnessed, and all the many ways we can make change.

Dr. Blumenthal is a great example of this. She saw the need for public-private partnerships that could further women's health initiatives, so she called up the Girl Scouts of America and encouraged them to make women's health a focal point of what they teach young girls. They worked together on a smoking prevention badge that was announced at the White House. She also contacted producers and scriptwriters and asked them to weave women's health issues into their scripts.

Or look at Tiffany. She lives in Virginia, and in 2025 she and the ACR applied for a gubernatorial proclamation to recognize Lung Cancer Awareness month every November. The state accepted it! She also created National Lung Cancer Screening Day in 2021, and in 2025, I got to help celebrate its fourth anniversary. When I talked to her in November, Tiffany was in the midst of the busiest time of her year. She'd just finished lobbying radiology clinics to stay open on Saturdays so that people who work Monday through Friday and normally wouldn't have the opportunity to get screened could come in.

"We had close to 700 facilities pledge this year," Tiffany said. "I created this day to reduce stigma and celebrate the patients that are going to get screened. [At the centers I visited] it was like a party. I had white balloons. I ordered breakfast. I had T-shirts that said National Lung Cancer Screening Day and pins that said, 'I got screened' or 'Ask me about lung screening.' And these patients loved it. They're like, 'I used to get so nervous because I thought I was going to get yelled at coming in for a screening, and you just made it a celebration.'"

Fighting lung cancer and advocating for increased screening feels like a ground-level game even at the best of times. When I asked Tiffany what she did last week, her answer showed just how scrappy lung cancer advocates like her are:

> The ACR has an effective economics and government relations team. There was this big uproar literally last Friday about the GO296 code, and that's the shared decision-making code that doctors have to submit along with the lung cancer screening code. If that code is not submitted, then the lung screening can't be done. During COVID, the CMS made it okay to do these doctor-patient discussions by televisit, making it easier for patients. Well, last Friday, CMS came out for some reason and said, oh, effective October 1, unless a patient is in a rural location, shared decision-making will not be covered if it was done via telemedicine. Well,

> that's a problem because these patients, who are at high risk for lung cancer and eligible for screening, may choose not to have these doctor-patient discussions, and then can't be screened. Big, big deal. I got on the phone and we got it fixed.

All of the people I've met inspire me daily. They motivate me to do everything I've done and everything I'll do in the future. I hope they inspire you, too.

Australia: A Model of Success

I've spent this entire book writing about the state of lung cancer detection and treatment in America, but I find it helpful to look at what other countries are doing to improve screening rates. I recently met Catherine Jones, a professor, cardiothoracic radiologist, AI developer, and radiology researcher based in Brisbane, Australia. Three and a half years ago, she was tasked with designing the National Lung Cancer Screening Program in Australia, and it launched on July 1, 2025.

Before 2025, Australia didn't have a lung cancer screening program. Today, if you are between fifty and seventy and have smoked the equivalent of thirty pack years, you are eligible for a fully paid screening, and that's due to the hard work of Professor Jones and her colleagues who designed the program.

(Continued . . .)

I was initially surprised to hear that Australia's eligibility guidelines were stricter than those in the United States, but Professor Jones assured me that the fact that it's a national, centrally implemented and deployed program, funded through their public health system, has made all the difference in its success rate. Instead of relying on individual insurers, hospitals, or organizations to manage screening, one body does it.

The goals of the screening program are threefold:

1. Reduce the mortality of lung cancer. Like in the United States, it's the deadliest cancer in Australia.
2. Smoking cessation. The program provides consultation about how to quit smoking.
3. Reach the most vulnerable, high-risk populations. Professor Jones explained that many Australians who live in remote areas—particularly Indigenous Australians, non-native English speakers, disabled people, and members of the LGBTQ+ community—are more likely to have poor outcomes when they are diagnosed with lung cancer.

Six months into the program, the results have been nothing short of phenomenal. In fact, Australia is well on the way to surpassing the dismal 18 percent screening rate in the United States.

"Across Australia, there's just under a million eligible people who could be scanned," said Professor Jones.

"And we all thought, well, we can't do a million people in the first year. That's ridiculous. . . .So we were expecting somewhere between, say, 100,000 and 200,000 people in the first year. But that was a really optimistic projection, because that's ten to twenty percent of eligible people in the first year. The US program hasn't even achieved nineteen percent and they've been doing this for more than ten years. Well, we've just cracked our 40,000th person without advertising to the public . . . we're not actually even halfway through the year. So I think realistically, we're going to do more than 100,000 scans in the first year."

Australia has a central registry for cancer screening, so they're able to integrate the lung cancer program into that existing registry to enable all the data to be collected centrally. In America, ACR has a similar program, but it's not government-mandated, and providers have to pay money to upload their results. (Most providers just don't have the staff or money for this kind of work.) Secondly, they have made significant direct appeals to primary care physicians, who've gobbled up the information and started scanning their patient lists to see who might be eligible. The screening program provides educational material to doctors, radiologists, and technicians about how to approach that conversation with empathy and kindness in order to reduce the stigma around smoking. As in America, Australia wants to change the image of

(Continued . . .)

lung cancer patients from a grizzled old man with yellow fingers and a cigarette between his lips to someone like me: in my forties, female, and a never-smoker.

The media also took notice, and the program has been promoted far and wide on Australian TV and in newspapers. Finally, they've deployed a mobile screening unit to reach Australians in remote areas with money from the government to build five more. "They're these great big double semi-trailers," Professor Jones told me, "with two massive units on the back of it and branding all over, saying 'come and get your lungs looked at,' Everybody wants to come and have a bit of a look at it because it's, you know, *ooh*. And the older men in town are like, 'I might go and have a look because that looks like good engineering.'"

The screening program has an additional aim: to gather data on family history to demonstrate that people with a close relative with lung cancer are more likely to develop it themselves. Professor Jones estimates she has data on about five thousand cases so far, and when she and her team review the program in two years' time, she hopes to expand the screening guidelines to include people with a first-degree relative history of primary lung cancer.

"There's a whole bunch of other criteria that we are working on generating the evidence for," Professor Jones adds. "For example, people who work in occupational exposed workplaces, particularly those who've been exposed historically to asbestos or mine dust disease. . . . And then there's the women. So just like you, Shira, women who have never smoked, we know that the incidence of lung cancer in that group is rising year after year. We don't really know why, but we know that that is the biggest untapped group of lung cancer patients out there."

Professor Jones very much wants to avoid the situation I faced: presenting with a nodule on a scan and then being told I should come back only if I had symptoms. "If they don't fit that textbook example of someone who's a chain smoker," she said, "they get told, 'oh, look, it's not going to be anything to worry about. Come back in a few months. Yeah, or it's probably just a minor infection, you'll get over it.' And they don't plan to do anything else about it."

Will the screening age go down as well? Professor Jones feels sure that it will.

"So, all of the major screening trials around the world usually start at age fifty-five," she said. "We decided to make it fifty because we know that particularly in our Indigenous community, the spike really happens between fifty and fifty-five. I can see a possibility of reducing that entrance age to say forty-five for people who might be Indigenous or who have a family history. That's the next easy step to take because the evidence is starting to show that already. We do things that are pretty much evidence based. So there's a flurry of research activity happening

(Continued . . .)

over the last few years to generate evidence in order to be able to justify essentially the extra cost of screening people in those extra age groups as well as the extra eligibility criteria."

I admire what Professor Jones and her country are doing beyond anything I can describe. She's finding people who are eligible for screening and making it easy for them to get scanned. Her appeals to doctors have worked, and the education has started to reach the masses.

If Australia can do it, so can we! We are now just on the cusp of finding new and effective ways of screening more people for lung cancer. New blood tests are under development that will hopefully supplement LDCTs as well.

Afterword

In January 2025, before my diagnosis, I went to a gift exchange with a few of my girlfriends. We drank wine and ate tiny cookies, sharing stories about our kids and our husbands and laughing at all the adventures we'd had over the last year. Midway through the party, we pulled our chairs into a circle, and we went around the room one by one, telling everyone where we saw ourselves at the end of the year. I was *so* glad I was one of the last people called on because I really wasn't sure what to say. Like so many moms, almost everything I do in my life is in service to my family, sometimes at the expense of my own self-care. Sure, I have running, a job I love, and a ton of friends who'd do almost anything for me, but, all too often, my priorities center on other people.

"I'm not looking for a *passion* this year," I said when it was finally my turn. "I just want to figure out my purpose. What is it I'm here to do? What can I do to really assert my self-worth?"

I didn't find my purpose, but when I got lung cancer, it found me. This illness has been the hardest pill I've ever swallowed, but I'm so grateful for all I've learned from it and everyone I've met because of it. I may have spent the month of October in doctors' appointments, inside a scanner, under a surgeon's knife, or lying on my back porch, trying not to put any pressure on my right side, but it was all worth it. I always suspected I had a mission in the world, I just didn't know what it was. Now I do.

In early November, I flew to Washington, DC with Adam, Eric, and Kim for a few Lung Cancer Awareness Month events. While I was there, I met Tiffany for the first time, as well as many other lung cancer experts and advocates whose names I haven't mentioned in this book. I bought a white suit, put on my white ribbon, and stepped off the plane as excited as my kids were when Taylor Swift came to town. In Washington, I'd be with *my people*, the lung cancer warriors. We knew what kind of monster we were up against, but we had the knowledge, will, and determination to battle against it.

On November 3, 2025, LUNGevity, a nonprofit dedicated to research, education, and support for lung diseases, planted sixty thousand white flags in the National Mall, with each one representing two lives lost to lung cancer each year. The day was picture perfect, with blue skies and mild temperatures, and the flags stretched on for yards, fluttering in unison when a breeze blew through. As I stood facing them, I realized I've never felt so humbled. Those flags stood for human lives that had been snuffed out too soon. They were people with children, spouses, pets, friends, jobs, and hobbies. They had hopes, dreams, failures, and life lessons they'd learned on the way. Each one of those people, like me, also had no idea that a cancer was growing inside them. They likely endured treatments that were meant to extend their lives rather than save them, and that's a tragedy. If they'd had access to early screening, they might have lived. I knew, deep in my heart, that it was a miracle that I wasn't among them. I'm a lung cancer survivor, and that's a rarity.

"Another thing that I've been working on is survivorship, making more survivorship," said Tiffany a few weeks after we'd returned home from Washington, while I was researching this book. "I want to show that, hey, you can survive lung cancer. It is not a death sentence anymore."

Looking out over those sixty thousand flags, I hoped for a day where we could plant sixty thousand flags for all the lives saved. Because lung cancer doesn't have to be a killer. It hasn't been for me, and it doesn't have to be for you, either.

Today, we can redouble our research efforts, including identifying blood test biomarkers, pinpointing risk factors, and developing new, innovative screening techniques as well as treatments. But, unfortunately, until we get people through the doors of a radiology clinic or mobile unit, we'll never catch lung cancer early enough to make treatment simple. Unless you take a few hours out of your busy life and lie inside a shiny tube, you'll never know if a bundle of cells inside your lungs is growing into cancer.

My mission is to spread the word about early screening and urge you and your loved ones to do it if you feel you're at risk. Even if you aren't, consider getting a scan just to be sure. It's so easy! All it takes is an hour and a set of lungs. One scan saved my life, and that should be the case for you, too.

Acknowledgments

Sitting down to write this book has brought such a wide range of emotions. It has given me the ability to really pause and process what my life has looked like these last few months. The initial fears of "I have what?" and "how could this happen to me?" were put on the back burner as I defended myself and my lifestyle to those closest to me. I was forced to confront the narrative that lung cancer is a "deserved disease." That all my careful life choices—all the healthy meals, always turning down a cigarette, the miles and miles I ran each day—none of them mattered. Lung cancer still found me, and it will find many others who have tried their hardest to hide from it too.

This journey has also proven to me the power of community. I have found endless inspiration from those around me, and those I have been introduced to during this season. I found that I am an oversharer. I run to tell the world about my diagnosis only to find so many other survivors keeping their lips sealed. I have worked with many of them to share their stories as well as quietly supporting those who wish to still keep it a secret. Thank you to the survivors, Erik Hale, Donnita Butler, and Heidi Onda, who contributed to my book and were strong enough to come forward. Thank you to Skyhorse Publishing, especially Tony Lyons and Daniela Rapp, for believing in me and also to Sarah Durand for helping me to write my own story.

Thank you to my husband, the bulldozer, who cried alone during my diagnosis on a plane from Afghanistan to Qatar and who pushed me through my cancer journey in just one week's time. I love my parents, both doctors, who I have listened to my whole life, who were there every step of the way to explain the confusing nuances of my diagnosis. Adam's parents also came to help nurture me and play with the kids. My siblings, Adam's siblings, my friends, and colleagues all came running with flowers, cozy jammies and warm soups. Really, my people and my team and my community were amazing! I appreciate my dear friend Kim, and her father, who fought for me, took me seriously, and encouraged me to get to the other side. Thank you to Dr. Grogan, who so thoughtfully and thoroughly answered my every question—and actually cut out my cancer! Many thanks to Dr. Lentz, who met me at the start of it all and walked me through the entire process. And of course, to Dr. Osterman and all of the other oncologists who hold my hand through the future decisions on which medications to use or not to use. I am able to share my story because they were able to get me to today.

I have been so inspired by the conversations I have had with teams of people at the preeminent scanning businesses, the current and past government administrations, and health insurance companies. Dr. Mehmet Oz answered my call the day of my diagnosis. He gave sound advice not just as the current Medicare and Medicaid Administrator but also as a seasoned world-renowned thoracic surgeon. He guided me through the surgery and sat with me to listen during recovery. Secretary Kennedy and Stephanie Spear showed me that prevention is not a partisan issue, it is an American issue. The Aetna CEO and CMO listened as I helped change their perspective on lung cancer and the facts surrounding the truth behind it not being a lifestyle choice disease. To strong CEOs like Anne Wojcicki, who lost her sister to cancer, who was raised by a wonderful mother that lost a daughter and who will never be forgotten. I am confident that we will be able to work together to make sure my story is possible and affordable and accessible for all Americans.

Thank you to all the experts who lent their years of knowledge and passion for advocacy to this book, including Dr. Susan Blumenthal, Professor Catherine Jones, and Tiffany Gowen. This book would not have been possible without you.

My journey has proven to me that there is a larger force at play. That this whole process may actually be *beshert*, meant to be, kismet. Though Lung Cancer Survivor was not a life goal I hoped for, it has opened my eyes to a larger meaning in life and helped guide me today. It is time to change the narrative on lung cancer, and it is time to take control of our own health and be proactive with our care. Thank you to all the lung cancer survivors, loved ones, and advocates who have paved the way to make this happen.

Notes

Introduction

1 R. L. Siegel, K. D. Miller, H. E. Fuchs, A. Jemal, "Cancer statistics, 2022," *CA Cancer J Clin.*, 2022;72:7–33.
2 M. C. DeRouen et al., "Integrating Electronic Health Record, Cancer Registry, and Geospatial Data to Study Lung Cancer in Asian American, Native Hawaiian, and Pacific Islander Ethnic Groups," *Cancer Epidemiol Biomarkers,* Prev. 2021, Aug;30(8):1506–16. doi: 10.1158/1055-9965.EPI-21-0019. Epub 2021 May 17. PMID: 34001502; PMCID: PMC8530225.
3 National Lung Screening Trial Research Team et al., "The National Lung Screening Trial: overview and study design," *Radiology* 258,1 (2011):243–53. doi:10.1148/radiol.10091808

Chapter 2

1 David S Gierada, et al., "Low-Dose CT Screening for Lung Cancer: Evidence from 2 Decades of Study," *Radiology. Imaging Cancer* 2,2 e190058. 27 Mar. 2020, doi:10.1148/rycan.2020190058.
2 Takeshi Kubo, et al., "Standard-dose vs. low-dose CT protocols in the evaluation of localized lung lesions: Capability for lesion characterization-iLEAD study," *European Journal of Radiology Open,* 367–73. 24 Mar. 2016, doi:10.1016/j.ejro.2016.03.002.

Chapter 3

1 C. I. Henschke et al., "International Early Lung Cancer Action Program Investigators. A 20-year Follow-up of the International Early Lung Cancer Action Program (I-ELCAP)," *Radiology,* 2023 Nov;309(2):e231988. doi: 10.1148/radiol.231988. PMID: 37934099; PMCID: PMC10698500.
2 A. W. Maiga et al., "Mapping Histoplasma capsulatum Exposure, United States," *Emerging Infectious Diseases,* 2018;24(10):1835–39. doi:10.3201/eid2410.180032.

Chapter 4

1 K. Song et al., "A quantitative method for assessing smoke associated molecular damage in lung cancers," *Transl Lung Cancer Res.,*

2018 Aug;7(4):439–49. doi: 10.21037/tlcr.2018.07.01. PMID: 30225209; PMCID: PMC6131178.

2 U.S. Department of Health and Human Services, *Smoking Cessation. A Report of the Surgeon General,* Atlanta, GA: U.S. Department of Health and Human Services, Centers for Disease Control and Prevention, National Center for Chronic Disease Prevention and Health Promotion, Office on Smoking and Health, 2020. [accessed 2022 Feb 7].

3 Office on Smoking and Health (US), "The Health Consequences of Involuntary Exposure to Tobacco Smoke: A Report of the Surgeon General," Atlanta (GA): Centers for Disease Control and Prevention (US); 2006.

4 U.S. Dept of Health and Human Services, "The Health Consequences of Smoking—50 Years of Progress: A Report of the Surgeon General," U.S. Dept of Health and Human Services; 2014.

5 M. P. Rivera et al., "Lung Cancer Screening in Cancer Survivors vs Those Without a History of Cancer," *JAMA Netw Open.*, 2025 Sep 2;8(9):e2535000. doi: 10.1001/jamanetworkopen.2025.35000. PMID: 41026483; PMCID: PMC12485636.

6 Y. G. Lee et al., "Assessment of Lung Cancer Risks Related to Family History in Never-Smokers: A Cohort Study," *Clin Lung Cancer,* 2025 Jul;26(5):364–69.e2. doi: 10.1016/j.cllc.2025.04.003. Epub 2025 Apr 8. PMID: 40348730.

Chapter 5

1 A. Jemal et al. "The Burden of Lung Cancer in Women Compared With Men in the US." *JAMA Oncol.* 2023;9(12):1727–28. oi:10.1001/jamaoncol.2023.4415

2 S. L. Gomez et al., "Elevated risk of lung cancer among Asian American women who have never smoked: an emerging cancer disparity," *J Natl Cancer Inst.*, 2025 Jun 1;117(6):1104–9. doi: 10.1093/jnci/djae299. PMID: 39565906.

3 Elaine Shum et al., "Preliminary results from the Female Asian Nonsmoker Screening Study (FANSS)," *J Clin Oncol* 41, 8510(2023). DOI:10.1200/JCO.2023.41.16_suppl.8510.

4 Yue-Lun Zhang, et al., "The prevalence of EGFR mutation in patients with non-small cell lung cancer: a systematic review and meta-analysis," *Oncotarget* 7,48 (2016):78985–93. doi:10.18632/oncotarget.12587.

5 A. M. Chapman et al., "Lung cancer mutation profile of EGFR, ALK, and KRAS: meta-analysis and comparison of never and ever smokers," *Lung Cancer,* 102 (2016), 122–34.

6 A. Midha, S. Dearden, R. McCormack, "EGFR mutation incidence in non-small-cell lung cancer of adenocarcinoma histology: a systematic review and global map by ethnicity (mutMapII)," *Am J Cancer Res*, 5 (2015):2892.

7 G. C. Chang et al., "TALENT Investigators. Low-dose CT screening among never-smokers with or without a family history of lung cancer in Taiwan: a prospective cohort study," *Lancet Respir Med.*, 2024 Feb;12(2):141–52. doi: 10.1016/S2213-2600(23)00338-7. Epub 2023 Nov 29. PMID: 38042167.

8 National Institutes of Health. (2022). NIH Clinical Center Data Report. (NIH Publication Number 22-8004). U.S. Department of Health and Human Services, National Institutes of Health. Retrieved January 22, 2026, https://www.cc.nih.gov/sites/default/files/assets/about/pdf/2022CCDataReport.pdf

Chapter 7

1 Centers for Disease Control and Prevention. National Center for Health Statistics. National Health Interview Survey, 1965-2022. Analysis performed by the American Lung Association Epidemiology and Statistics Unit using SPSS software.

2 National Lung Screening Trial Research Team: D. R. Aberle, A. M. Adams, C. D. Berg, W. C. Black, J. D. Clapp, R. M. Fagerstrom, I. F. Gareen, C. Gatsonis, P. M. Marcus, J. D. Sicks, "Reduced lung-cancer mortality with low-dose computed tomographic screening," *N Engl J Med.*, 2011 Aug 4;365(5):395–409. doi: 10.1056/NEJMoa1102873. Epub 2011 Jun 29. PMID: 21714641; PMCID: PMC4356534.

3 M. C. Aldrich et al., "Evaluation of USPSTF Lung Cancer Screening Guidelines Among African American Adult Smokers," *JAMA Oncol.*, 2019 Sep 1;5(9):1318–24. doi: 10.1001/jamaoncol.2019.1402. Erratum in: *JAMA Oncol.* 2019 Sep 1;5(9):1372. doi: 10.1001/jamaoncol.2019.3296. PMID: 31246249; PMCID: PMC6604090.

4 American Lung Association. "State of Lung Cancer (2022)." Available at: https://www.lung.org/research/state-of-lung-cancer/key-findings

5 M. Siahpush, G. H. Singh, P. R. Jones, L. R. Timsina, "Racial/Ethnic and Socioeconomic Variations in Duration of Smoking: Results from 2003, 2006 and 2007 Tobacco Use Supplement of the Current Population Survey," *Journal of Public Health*, 2009;32(2):210.

6 Centers for Disease Control and Prevention. National Center for Health Statistics. *National Health Interview Survey, 2023*. Analysis performed by the American Lung Association Epidemiology and Statistics Unit using SPSS software.
7 Sources for smoke-free states, cities and counties: American Nonsmokers' Rights Foundation, https://nosmoke.org/wp-content/uploads/pdf/SummaryUSPopList.pdf; http://www.no-smoke.org/pdf/EffectivePopulationList.pdf. Accessed July 7, 2025.
8 Julia M Coughlin, et al., "Understanding barriers to lung cancer screening in primary care." *Journal of Thoracic Disease* 12,5 (2020):2536–44. doi:10.21037/jtd.2020.03.66.

Chapter 8

1 J. Allen-Dicker, A. Auerbach, S. J. Herzig, "Perceived Safety and Value of Inpatient 'Very Important Person' Services," *J Hosp Med.,* 2017 Mar;12(3):177–79. doi: 10.12788/jhm.2701. PMID: 28272595.
2 D. Kim, W. Woo, J. I. Shin, S. Lee, "The Uncomfortable Truth: Open Thoracotomy versus Minimally Invasive Surgery in Lung Cancer: A Systematic Review and Meta-Analysis," *Cancers* (Basel), 2023 May 5;15(9):2630. doi: 10.3390/cancers15092630. PMID: 37174096; PMCID: PMC10177030.
3 J. M. Pan et al., "The Surgical Renaissance: Advancements in Video-Assisted Thoracoscopic Surgery and Robotic-Assisted Thoracic Surgery and Their Impact on Patient Outcomes," *Cancers* (Basel), 2024 Sep 5;16(17):3086. doi: 10.3390/cancers16173086. PMID: 39272946; PMCID: PMC11393871.

Chapter 9

1 M. Simon, K. Zukotynski, D. M. Naeger, "Pulmonary nodules as incidental findings," *CMAJ*, 2018 Feb 12;190(6):E167. doi: 10.1503/cmaj.171223. PMID: 29440337; PMCID: PMC5809217.
2 P. J. Mazzone and L. Lam, "Evaluating the Patient with a Pulmonary Nodule: A Review," *JAMA,* 2022 Jan 18;327(3):264–73. doi: 10.1001/jama.2021.24287. PMID: 35040882.

Chapter 10

1 American Lung Association. (2025). State of Lung Cancer. Retrieved January 22,2026 from https://www.lung.org/getmedia/5f587b49-4f94-4fd0-8e57-c55de5e684b5/SOLC-2025-Print-Report.pdf.

Chapter 11

1 T. Nyberg, D. Frost, D. Barrowdale, D. G. Evans, E. Bancroft , J. Adlard, M. Ahmed, J. Barwell, A. F. Brady, C. Brewer, J. Cook,

R. Davidson,A. Donaldson, J. Eason, H. Gregory, A. Henderson, L. Izatt, M. J. Kennedy, C. Miller, P. J. Morrison, A. Murray, K. R. Ong, M. Porteous, C. Pottinger, M. T. Rogers, L. Side, K. Snape, L. Walker, M. Tischkowitz, R. Eeles, D. F. Easton, A. C. Antoniou. Prostate Cancer Risks for Male BRCA1 and BRCA2 Mutation Carriers: A Prospective Cohort Study. *Eur Urol.* 2020 Jan;77(1):24–35.

2 Vivek Mittal. 2018. Epithelial Mesenchymal Transition in Tumor Metastasis. *Annual Review Pathology: Mechanisms Disease.* 13:395–412. https://doi.org/10.1146/annurev-pathol-020117-043854

3 H. A. Yu et al., "Germline EGFR T790M mutation found in multiple members of a familial cohort," *J Thorac Oncol.,* 2014;9(4):554–58. doi: 10.1097/JTO.0000000000000052.

4 Geoffrey R. Oxnard et al., "Germline *EGFR* Mutations and Familial Lung Cancer," *J Clin Oncol* 41, 5274–84(2023). DOI:10.1200/JCO.23.01372.

5 M. C. Aldrich et al., "Evaluation of USPSTF Lung Cancer Screening Guidelines Among African American Adult Smokers," *JAMA Oncol.,* 2019;5(9):1318–24. doi:10.1001/jamaoncol.2019.1402

6 D. Schrag et al., "Blood-based tests for multicancer early detection (PATHFINDER): a prospective cohort study," *Lancet,* 2023 Oct 7;402(10409):1251–60. doi: 10.1016/S0140-6736(23)01700-2. PMID: 37805216; PMCID: PMC11027492.

Chapter 12

1 M. Boubnovski Martell et al., "Radiomics for lung cancer diagnosis, management, and future prospects," *Clinical Radiology* 86, 106926.

Chapter 13

1 M. E. Arcila, et al., "EGFR exon 20 insertion mutations in lung adenocarcinomas: prevalence, molecular heterogeneity, and clinicopathologic characteristics," *Mol. Cancer Ther.* 12, 220–29 (2013).

Chapter 14

1 Mario Mascalchi and Lapo Sali, "Lung cancer screening with low dose CT and radiation harm-from prediction models to cancer incidence data," *Annals of Translational Medicine* 5,17 (2017): 360. doi:10.21037/atm.2017.06.41.

2 H. C. Yang et al., "Age-Based Screening for Lung Cancer Surveillance in the US," *JAMA Netw Open.,* 2025 Nov 3;8(11):e2546222. doi: 10.1001/jamanetworkopen.2025.46222. PMID: 41264266; PMCID: PMC12635884.

Chapter 15

1 P. Bandi et al., "Lung Cancer Deaths Prevented and Life-Years Gained from Lung Cancer Screening," *JAMA*, 2025 Nov 19;334(24):2225–27. doi: 10.1001/jama.2025.19798. Epub ahead of print. PMID: 41259039; PMCID: PMC12631561.

2 P. D. Joshi, C. J. Wakslak, G. Appel, and L. Huang, (2020) "Gender differences in communicative abstraction," *J. Personal. Soc. Psychol.,* 118, 417–35. doi: 10.1037/pspa0000177.

3 S. Matoff-Stepp, B. Applebaum, J. Pooler, E. Kavanagh, "Women as health care decision-makers: implications for health care coverage in the United States," *J Health Care Poor Underserved*, 2014 Nov;25(4):1507–13. doi: 10.1353/hpu.2014.0154. PMID: 25418222.

4 Yan Wang, et al., "Risk and Influencing Factors for Subsequent Primary Lung Cancer After Treatment of Breast Cancer: A Systematic Review and Two Meta-Analyses Based on Four Million Cases," *Journal of Thoracic Oncology* 16(11):1893–1908.

5 K. L. Sandler et al., "Women screened for breast cancer are dying from lung cancer: An opportunity to improve lung cancer screening in a mammography population," *J Med Screen.*, 2021 Dec;28(4):488–93. doi: 10.1177/09691413211013058. Epub 2021 May 4. PMID: 33947284.

6 Jani Chinmay et al., "CALM: Coordinating a Lung Screening with Mammography," *CHEST* 164(4):A3998–A3999.

7 Robert J. Fortuna et al., "A Comprehensive, Multidisciplinary Approach to Improving Lung Cancer Screening," *NEJM Catalyst*, 2025;6(11). DOI: 10.1056/CAT.25.0051.

8 H. C. Yang et al., "Age-Based Screening for Lung Cancer Surveillance in the US," *JAMA Netw Open.*, 2025;8(11):e2546222. doi:10.1001/jamanetworkopen.2025.46222.

9 Surveillance Research Program, National Cancer Institute, "Breast Cancer—Long-term trends in SEER age-adjusted mortality rates, 1975–2023, by sex, all races, all ages," SEER*Explorer. Accessed on April 17, 2025. https://seer.cancer.gov/explorer/, 2025.

10 K. S. Almberg et al., "Increased odds of mortality from non-malignant respiratory disease and lung cancer are highest among US coal miners born after 1939," *Occup Environ Med.*, 2023 Mar;80(3):121–28. doi: 10.1136/oemed-2022-108539. Epub 2023 Jan 12. PMID: 36635098; PMCID: PMC10428099.